Hypnosis for Chronic Pain Management

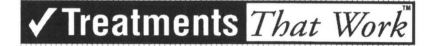

Hypnosis for Chronic Pain Management

Workbook

Mark P. Jensen

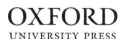
OXFORD
UNIVERSITY PRESS

UNIVERSITY PRESS

Oxford University Press, Inc., publishes works that further
Oxford University's objective of excellence
in research, scholarship, and education.

Oxford   New York
Auckland   Cape Town   Dar es Salaam   Hong Kong   Karachi
Kuala Lumpur   Madrid   Melbourne   Mexico City   Nairobi
New Delhi   Shanghai   Taipei   Toronto

With offices in
Argentina   Austria   Brazil   Chile   Czech Republic   France   Greece
Guatemala   Hungary   Italy   Japan   Poland   Portugal   Singapore
South Korea   Switzerland   Thailand   Turkey   Ukraine   Vietnam

Published by Oxford University Press, Inc.
198 Madison Avenue, New York, New York 10016
www.oup.com

Oxford is a registered trademark of Oxford University Press

ISBN-13 978-0-19-977238-4 (Paper)

9 8 7 6 5 4 3 2 1

Printed in the United States of America

About Treatments *ThatWork*™

One of the most difficult problems confronting patients with various disorders and diseases is finding the best help available. Everyone is aware of friends or family who have sought treatment from a seemingly reputable practitioner, only to find out later from another doctor that the original diagnosis was wrong or the treatments recommended were inappropriate or perhaps even harmful. Most patients, or family members, address this problem by reading everything they can about their symptoms, seeking out information on the Internet, or aggressively "asking around" to tap knowledge from friends and acquaintances. Governments and healthcare policymakers are also aware that people in need don't always get the best treatments—something they refer to as "variability in healthcare practices."

Now healthcare systems around the world are attempting to correct this variability by introducing "evidence-based practice." This simply means that it is in everyone's interest that patients get the most up-to-date and effective care for a particular problem. Healthcare policymakers have also recognized that it is very useful to give consumers of health care as much information as possible, so that they can make intelligent decisions in a collaborative effort to improve health and mental health. This series, Treatments *That Work*™, is designed to accomplish just that. Only the latest and most effective interventions for particular problems are described, in user-friendly language. To be included in this series, each treatment program must pass the highest standards of evidence available, as determined by a scientific advisory board. Thus, when individuals suffering from these problems or their family members seek out an expert clinician who is familiar with these interventions and decides that they are appropriate, they will have confidence that they are receiving the best care available. Of course, only your healthcare professional can decide on the right mix of treatments for you.

This workbook is written for people with chronic pain who want to turn their lives around, and are interested in learning how to use self-hypnosis to help them achieve this. Whether you suffer from headaches, back pain, nerve damage, or pain caused by disability, trauma, or injury, this workbook can help.

You may have been invited to read this book by your clinician who plans to teach you self-hypnosis skills for feeling better, sleeping better, and doing more. Or you might be reading this book because you are curious about how you might use self-hypnosis to learn how to better manage your pain. Regardless of how you came upon this book, you can use it successfully to manage your pain problems.

Part I includes educational materials about pain and the biology of pain. Part II helps you understand more about hypnosis and how it can help with pain, and Part III presents instructions for self-hypnosis that you can use to accomplish your goals of lessening pain, improving mood, and enhancing sleep.

The hypnosis treatment described in this book, and that you could receive from your clinician, has been scientifically tested and found to be effective for reducing the intensity of chronic pain. It will teach you skills for pain management that you can use at any time, and for the rest of your life.

David H. Barlow, Editor-in-Chief,
Treatments *ThatWork*™
Boston, MA

This book is dedicated to the relief of pain and suffering.

Acknowledgments

The information and advice presented in this book come, in large part, from many hours of training, encouragement, and advice that I received from two colleagues: Drs. Joseph Barber and David R. Patterson. Their work and contributions continue to inspire me.

The book also benefited greatly from the editorial assistance of Lisa C. Murphy, whose thoughtful advice helped to keep the material clear.

The book could not have been written without the financial support for the research studies that provided the findings supporting the procedures described in the workbook. Funding from the National Institutes of Health (National Center for Medical Rehabilitation Research), the Department of Education (National Institute on Disability and Rehabilitation Research), the Paralyzed Veterans of America, and the National Multiple Sclerosis Society, in particular, was key to building an understanding of the effects and efficacy of self-hypnosis training.

Finally, our research program studying hypnotic analgesia could not proceed without the many individuals with chronic pain who volunteer to participate as participants in the research supporting this work. Their willingness to share their experiences with the treatments described here has been essential for advancing knowledge in the field.

Contents

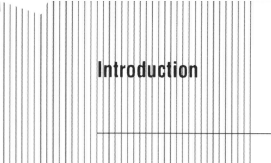

Introduction

Goals

■ To understand that chronic pain is common and can interfere with all aspects of your life

■ To understand that the medical treatments currently available for chronic pain are limited

■ To consider learning self-hypnosis skills so that you can get more control over pain and its effects on your life

Chronic Pain Is Common and Can Interfere with All Aspects of Your Life

If you are reading this workbook, then you probably have chronic pain, or know someone who does. You are not alone: between 70% and 90% of people have problems with headache at some point in their lives, and between 10% and 20% have chronic headache problems. Low back pain is even more common: 80% of the population has low back pain at some point in their lives, and close to 30% report having low back pain at any one time. Pain problems due to nerve damage (for example, from diabetes) are also very common. Chronic pain can also result from having a disability such as spinal cord injury, multiple sclerosis, acquired amputation, or muscular dystrophy. It can result from a traumatic accident or injury, such as an automobile accident or fall. Chronic pain can emerge after a surgery, or as a side effect of medical treatment, such as chemotherapy for cancer.

Not only is chronic pain common, but it can also interfere substantially with all aspects of a person's life. If you have chronic pain, it is likely that it interferes with your ability to get to sleep or stay asleep. Your pain may also interfere with your ability to work, or to engage in your favorite hobby. It may interfere with your ability to enjoy yourself with your friends and family. You may even feel like a completely different person now, compared to what you were like before you had chronic pain. You may get moody at times, especially when the pain is severe, and may feel helpless, hopeless, or depressed in the face of pain. If you have been unable to exercise or be active because of pain, you may have gained weight since the onset of your pain problem. This additional weight can put a burden on your muscles, ligaments, and joints, which can cause even more pain.

The Medical Treatments Currently Available for Chronic Pain Are Limited

If we can build satellite and computer communication networks, we should be able to find a cure for chronic pain, right? It should be a very simple thing to find the nerve that transmits pain from the damaged part of the body to the brain, and then cut that nerve so that you feel no pain, at least from that part of your body. It should be easy to find a drug that can stop or slow down the pain message, so that you can then get on with your life.

Unfortunately, it is not so easy. We will discuss later in this workbook how the brain and body create the experience of pain, and we will learn that pain is not as simple as it might appear. If you cut a nerve, for example, the brain can respond to the lack of input that results as an indication of physical damage, and then create a sensation of pain that is even more severe than the original pain was. *Surgery to treat pain alone has not been found to be effective, and in fact can make the pain problem worse.*

Also, there is no such thing as a "pain killer." Even the most powerful analgesics, such as opioids (fentanyl, methadone, oxymorphone, oxycodone, hydrocodone), decrease pain intensity by only about 30% on average, and only for some people. For many others, these drugs at best "take the edge off" pain. In addition, over time people can build a tolerance for the pain-relieving effects of these drugs, requiring them to take more and more to have the same effects. People do not, however, develop a tolerance for the side effects, which can include nausea, constipation, sleepiness (but not improved sleep), and difficulty breathing.

Although people with chronic pain should not give up hope that better and more effective medications and medical treatments with fewer side effects may eventually be found, at this point in time there is no a cure for chronic pain. The question is, what should you do in the meantime? It might be tempting to just give up—to retreat and lie down, doing everything possible to minimize activity and take larger and larger doses of more powerful analgesics to feel at least some relief.

Unfortunately, however, such a response to pain can actually make the problem worse. As the body becomes weaker from lack of movement or exercise, it takes less and less physical activity to cause pain flare-ups. Worse yet, just waiting for the pain to get better on its own, or continuing to search for a cure that does not yet exist, can make people feel helpless and depressed when attempts to find a cure fail. This is no way to live. What can you do?

Getting Control over Your Pain and its Effects on Your Life

This book is written for people with chronic pain who want to turn their lives around, and are interested in learning how to use self-hypnosis to help them achieve this. You may have been invited to read this book by your clinician who plans to teach you self-hypnosis skills for feeling better, sleeping better, and doing more. Or you might be reading this book because you are curious about how you might use self-hypnosis to learn how to better manage your pain.

The hypnosis treatment that is described in this book, and that you could receive from your clinician, has been scientifically tested and found to be effective for reducing the intensity of chronic pain. It will teach you skills for pain management that you can use at any time, and for the rest of your life.

This workbook is written to help you get the most out of hypnosis treatment. It will answer many of the questions you might have about pain and hypnosis. The first four chapters explain some basic facts about the biology of pain, the psychology of pain, the history of hypnosis, and how hypnosis works. These chapters will help you understand that hypnosis does not "magically" take away pain.

Instead, hypnosis changes how your brain deals with the information it receives from the body. As a result of these changes, you will feel less pain and more in control.

The last half of the workbook will describe how you can use self-hypnosis to accomplish your goals. Hypnosis, like all other pain treatments, rarely cures pain. However, research shows that *almost all patients who learn self-hypnosis skills benefit from this approach* and most continue to use self-hypnosis skills long after treatment is over. You could be one of these people.

Part I: Understanding Pain

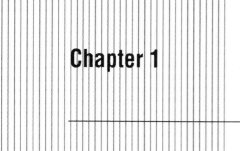

Chapter 1   *How Your Body and Brain Create Pain*

Goal

- To discover how the body and brain work together to create your experience of pain

Chapter Overview

To many people, hypnosis and self-hypnosis seem to work like "magic." Patients are often surprised that they feel so much pain relief during and after hypnosis sessions. At first, some might worry that because hypnosis worked so well for them, their pain may not be "real."

Rest assured that hypnosis works for "real" pain. This chapter summarizes what we know about the biological basis of pain, and lays the groundwork for you to understand how to use hypnosis to control your experience of pain. You do not have to read this chapter to benefit from hypnosis, but doing so may take away some of the mystery of how hypnosis works.

You will learn that the creation of a pain sensation is *not* simple. Many years ago, doctors thought that the brain was just a passive recipient of the sensory information from the body—that it received information about sights, smells, and other sensations like a TV that was stuck on one channel and one volume might receive a TV show. For such a TV, what you see, hear, and experience depends entirely on what is received. With this kind of TV, you have no control over what television show you see, or how loud the volume is.

We now know, however, that the brain works more like a fully functioning television. The brain can decide what channel to watch (the pain channel or the adventure channel?). Most importantly, perhaps, for our discussion, *the brain has a volume control knob and a channel changing knob that you can learn to use.*

The purpose of this chapter is to help you understand about how your brain's channel selector and volume controls work. It starts with a brief summary of the history of scientific theories of pain. It then describes how the *nerves* (the wires that send information from one part of the brain or body to another) work to create your experience of pain. The main message of this chapter is this: *Pain is the end result of activity in several different parts of your body and brain—you can therefore influence how much pain you feel by learning to get control over these processes.* Self-hypnosis is one way to do this.

How Your Body and Brain Work Together to Create Pain

In the 1600s, the French philosopher René Descartes argued that pain was a simple reflexive response to bodily injury. You drop a rock on your foot, you feel pain. The bigger the rock, the more pain you feel. A stubbed toe hurts less than a sprained ankle, which hurts less than a broken ankle. According to this model of pain, physical damage must always result in pain, and if you feel pain, there *must* be physical damage. And the more pain, the more the damage.

This view of pain was generally accepted by doctors and patients until the 1960s. Part of the reason for its wide acceptance is that the model seems to match our experience so closely. However, in hindsight, the flaws of this overly simplistic model become obvious. It does not explain, for example, how two people with the same amount of physical damage can experience different levels of pain. It does not explain some very real pain conditions where the patient can feel severe pain in response to very light touch. It also does not explain phantom limb pain, which occurs when a person feels pain in an amputated limb, foot, or hand that is no longer there. Descartes' outdated theory cannot explain how some athletes are able to continue to compete with broken bones or sprains during an intense game and not notice any pain until the game is over. These and many more examples tell us that Descartes' theory was too simplistic. Although physical damage to the body is *one factor* that can influence how much pain we feel, it turns out to be much less important than what the brain does with the information it receives.

In the 1960s, two scientists named Patrick Wall and Ronald Melzack found evidence that the amount of pain information going from the body to the brain is modified when it enters the spinal cord (the nerves that transmit information from the body to the brain enter the spinal cord at the "dorsal horn;" see Fig. 1.1). A "gate" at this location in the spinal cord can amplify or turn the volume down on the pain information that gets admitted into the spinal cord. For this reason, they called their model the "gate control theory" of pain. Importantly, they determined that the brain has control over the opening or closing of the gate. The gate lets more pain information into the spinal cord when a person is worried or anxious about pain, or spends time thinking about pain; the gate allows less pain information into the spinal cord when a person is focused on activities and thoughts unrelated to pain. For the first time, scientists had a biological explanation for why two people can have the same amount of physical damage, yet feel different amounts of pain. The model also gave us ideas about how people can change their thoughts and attention, and as a result feel less pain.

In the 40-plus years since the gate control theory was introduced, we have learned more about the way the brain responds to pain information from the body. We now know that a person will feel more or less pain *because of what the brain does with the information it receives.* This new understanding of pain explains why chronic pain treatments that focus only on the body part that hurts are not very effective. It also explains why treatments that focus on the brain, including hypnosis, can so effectively reduce pain for so many people.

Skin, Bones, and Muscle—the Periphery

Our skin, bones, and muscles contain sensors that respond to physical injury. When a body part is injured, these sensors send information towards the spinal cord. Depending on how open or closed the "gate" is in the spinal cord, more or less of this information about an injury will be allowed to reach the brain. The area of the body that contains these sensors lies outside of the brain and spinal cord and is called the *periphery* ("outer area"). The nerves that are embedded in these tissues are called peripheral nerves, and make up the peripheral

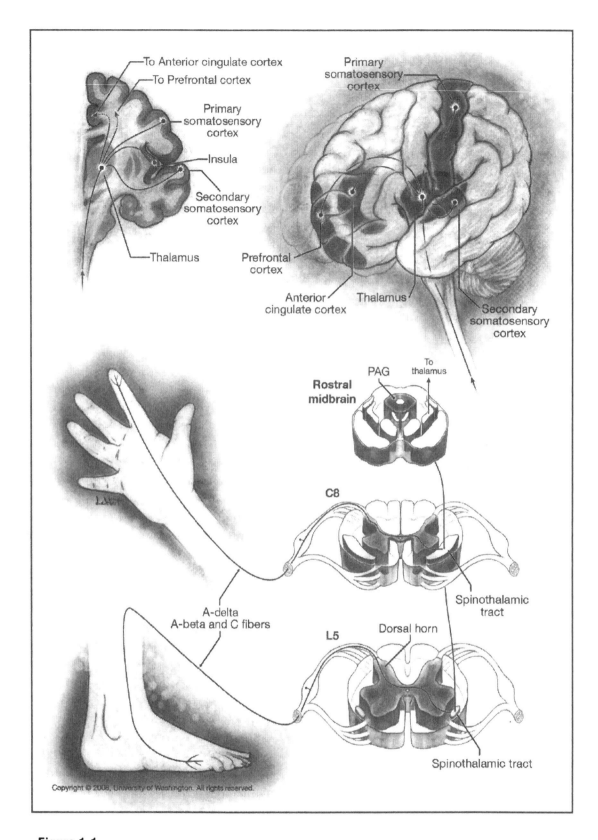

Labels in figure:

To Anterior cingulate cortex
To Prefrontal cortex
Primary somatosensory cortex
Insula
Secondary somatosensory cortex
Thalamus

Primary somatosensory cortex
Prefrontal cortex
Anterior cingulate cortex
Thalamus
Secondary somatosensory cortex

PAG
To thalamus
Rostral midbrain

C8

Spinothalamic tract

A-delta
A-beta and C fibers

L5
Dorsal horn

Spinothalamic tract

Figure 1.1

Primary peripheral and central nervous system components involved in the experience of pain nervous system. Nerves that lie within the spinal cord and brain make up the central nervous system.

The sensors in the peripheral tissues are connected to nerve fibers that send electrical signals to the spinal cord (see Fig. 1.1). The spinal cord is the highway that sends sensory information from the body to the brain. The nerve fibers that send most of the information about physical damage are of two types: (1) thin *C* fibers (thin because they do not have an insulating material covering them, which also makes them transmit information more slowly) and (2) thicker, insulated, and therefore faster, *A-delta* fibers. A third type, *A-beta*, normally carries information related to touch but can also transmit information that contributes to the experience of pain.

The Spinal Cord

The nerve fibers that send information about physical damage from the periphery to the brain enter the spine at the dorsal horn. However, the amount of information about pain that is allowed to get to the brain depends, in part, on whether the "gate" in the spinal cord is more open or more closed. As previously mentioned, being physically active and focused on non-pain activities, like an athlete in a game, tends to close the gate to pain messages. Being inactive and focused on or worried about pain tends to open the gate. Sometimes, people with chronic pain find that they are in a vicious cycle, where they become worried about pain and the brain responds by opening the pain gate and allowing more pain messages to be felt, which then increases pain further and makes the person more worried, which can then open the gate further, etc. As a result, the person feels more and more pain over time. To feel less pain, this cycle needs to be interrupted.

The Thalamus

Although the discussion so far has focused on the tissues and nerves outside of the brain, it is important to understand that information about physical damage arriving from the body by itself does not always produce pain. Pain is just a sensation until certain structures in the brain work together and become active. It is the brain that decides what sensations are pain and what sensations are not pain. It is the brain that decides how upset we are by those sensations. Importantly, *pain can be relieved when the structures and systems in the brain that create pain are interrupted.*

One of the brain structures that is active when we feel sensations is the *thalamus.* The thalamus is located right in the center of the brain. It is a kind of relay center that sends information from the spinal cord to other parts of the brain. The thalamus relays information that can potentially be turned into pain sensations directly to four other parts of the brain: (1) the *primary and secondary sensory cortices,* (2) the *insula,* (3) the *anterior cingulate cortex,* and (4) the *prefrontal cortex* (see Fig. 1.1).

Primary and Secondary Sensory Cortices

The *sensory cortex* is the part of the brain that works to tell us *where* we might be feeling a sensation (for example, the foot, head, belly, or hand) and how that sensation *feels* (for example, burning, cold, sharp, dull, or numb). The sensory cortex is divided into primary (S1) and secondary (S2) areas (see Fig. 1.1). Although the sensory cortex tells us the location and specific qualities of a sensation, it does not tell us how upsetting the pain is. It does not decide if we should do anything to stop the pain, or what the pain might mean to our lives. Other parts of the brain are needed for us to be upset about pain and to decide if we need to do something to relieve the pain.

Anterior Cingulate Cortex

The *anterior cingulate cortex* (ACC) lies between the two hemispheres of the brain (see Fig. 1.1). The ACC is involved in a large number of brain functions, including our emotional response to sensations and events. The ACC is very active when we are upset about pain, and calms down and become less active when we are not bothered by pain.

A very interesting study was recently performed that illustrates the importance of the ACC in our experience of pain. In this study, healthy individuals were taught how to gain control over activity in the ACC through biofeedback. To do this, they were put in a brain scanning machine and were given direct feedback about ACC activity. By being able to directly see the activity in their ACC, and with practice, they could learn to increase and decrease that activity. The most interesting finding from this study was that by changing ACC activity, the study subjects could change the intensity and unpleasantness of painful heat stimulation. When the stimulation occurred while the ACC was more active, the stimulation was rated as 23% more painful and 38% more unpleasant than when the ACC was less active. In other words, *the same amount of stimulation is felt as more or less painful due to the activity level in the ACC.* Moreover, people can learn to control this activity, and therefore control the level of pain. The stimulation and pain in this study were very "real." Yet the mind could be taught to control how intense that pain felt.

The scientists then taught a group of patients with chronic pain to decrease activity in the ACC using the same procedures. Note that the scientists did not do anything to the site of the patient's pain. They did not treat, fix, or cure any physical damage in these patients. They only taught the patients to alter activity in one part of the brain that needs to be active in order for a person to feel pain. The patients who received training reported a 44% decrease in the intensity of their chronic pain. The results of this study are consistent with what we now know about pain: *People can learn to get control over the severity of their pain by getting control over their brain activity.* Learning control over the ACC is one way to do this.

Insula

The *insula* lies deeply inside a fold of the brain, near the sensory cortex (see Fig. 1.1). The insula can be viewed as a kind of monitor for evaluating the body's overall health and well-being. The insula becomes active if and when the brain perceives that something is physically wrong—for example, if you need oxygen or food, or if the brain thinks that the body is physically damaged.

Prefrontal Cortex

The front surface of the brain (just behind your forehead) is called the *prefrontal cortex* (see Fig. 1.1). As it relates to pain, the prefrontal cortex processes memories about pain, the conclusions we make about the meaning that pain has in our lives, and the decisions we make about how we should cope with pain. In general, *more* activity in the prefrontal cortex is associated with less pain; the prefrontal cortex is important, therefore, for helping us to control pain.

Overall Brain Activity

So far, we have discussed very specific areas of the body and brain that are involved in the creation of a pain sensation. In addition to activity in these areas, scientists have also discovered that pain results in an overall increase in brain activity. It is as if, when someone is feeling pain, many different parts of the brain are talking all at once, like many people in a city panicking and screaming during an earthquake. Getting the brain to learn how to calm down, then, should result in an overall decrease in pain.

Long-Term Changes in Brain Activity with Chronic Pain

Finally, in addition to being associated with very focused (i.e., specific brain areas) and diffuse (across the whole brain) activity when we feel pain, ongoing chronic pain can cause longer-lasting physical changes in the brain. These changes affect how you will feel pain in the future. Unfortunately, these changes are not always positive. It is as if the brain learns to feel pain more easily, so that over time it takes less and less stimulation from the body to activate the brain areas that create pain.

Why It Is Important for You to Understand How the Body and Brain Create Pain

Understanding how the body and brain work together to create a pain sensation can help you in many ways. First, this knowledge can help you to understand why your pain does not always seem to be related to the amount of physical damage that is apparent to you and your doctor. You can have "good days" with less pain and "bad days" with more pain, even though there is no change in the physical state of the body part(s) that hurt. Chronic pain has much more to do with what the brain is doing with the information it receives than what is happening in skin, muscle, and bone. This does not mean that your pain is not "real;" *all pain is real.*

Based on what scientists have discovered about the biology of pain, it also makes sense that anything that results in changes in brain activity—and hypnosis does change brain activity (see Chapter 4)—can result in a decrease in your pain. This knowledge can give you hope—hope that when you learn to use self-hypnosis to directly alter activity in the sensory cortex, the ACC, insula, or prefrontal cortex, you will feel less pain. It also explains why so many people find that they experience pain relief when they practice self-hypnosis.

You do not have to give up hope for an *eventual* powerful medical treatment (or even cure) sometime in the future in order to learn to use hypnosis to help your pain now. Scientists are working very hard to find better treatments for chronic pain, and new discoveries are made every day. But what do you want to do in the meantime? One option is to learn some skills right now, today, to start to feel better. This workbook will help you get started to do this.

Chapter Summary

This chapter summarizes the current state-of-the-science understanding about the biological basis of pain. Descartes' theory of pain, developed roughly 350 years ago, argued that pain was merely a reflection of the amount of physical damage in our body. We now understand that pain is much more complicated than that. Although physical damage can influence the amount of pain we feel, the amount of physical damage is not the most important factor that affects how much pain we experience. Ultimately, it is the amount of activity in *different* areas of the brain that creates the sensation of pain. The primary generator of pain is the brain, and all of the pain we feel as a result of this process is very real.

The parts of the brain that play a role in the creation of pain are illustrated in Figure 1.1. They include those areas responsible for the meaning we give to pain (prefrontal cortex), the intensity and quality of pain (sensory cortices), the suffering component of pain (the ACC), and the extent to which the person judges that his or her body is physically at risk (the insula). These areas of the brain communicate with each other. Treatments that influence one area will affect activity in the other areas. This means that if you can learn to get control over some of these areas of the brain, for example, by using self-hypnosis to "calm" the brain, change how you think about pain, or change what your brain focuses on, you will feel less pain. The topic of this workbook is how you can use self-hypnosis to influence all of these areas, so that you can do more and hurt less.

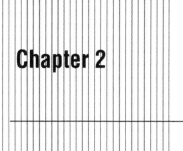

Chapter 2 How Thoughts and Coping Responses Influence Pain

Goals

- To understand how the thoughts you have about pain influence how you feel

- To identify the pain coping responses that can make you feel stronger and more comfortable

- To consider what changes you might want to make in your thoughts and coping responses so that you can do more and hurt less

Chapter Overview

The previous chapter described how the body and brain work together to create the experience of pain. This chapter will describe what scientists have discovered about the effects of your thoughts and coping responses on pain and your overall quality of life. Knowing this, you will be in a better position to discuss with your clinician and healthcare providers how you might want to change some of your pain-related thoughts and coping responses so that you can do more and hurt less.

Thoughts and Adjustment to Chronic Pain

Nancy is a 48-year-old woman who used to be very active. She loved sports, and played tennis in the summer and skied in the winter. She also enjoyed her job as the office manager of a family practice clinic. One weekend when she was doing some garden work she lifted a large bag of compost and heard a "pop" that sounded like it came from her low back. She also felt an immediate jabbing pain in her low back. She went to the emergency room and was told that she probably had "sprained a muscle or tendon" in her back, and that she should therefore rest in bed for a few days until she felt better.

But after seven days of resting, things did not get better. In fact, her pain only increased. Walking, bending, and sitting all made her back pain worse. In fact, just about any physical activity caused an increase in her pain. Her doctor recommended a scan of the back to determine if she had a ruptured disk in her spine. This test did not show a ruptured disk, although it did show that she had a "bulging" disk in her low back. Her doctor knew that bulging disks were very common in women of Nancy's age, and that bulging disks do not usually cause pain. He therefore could not say for certain if the bulging disk was the reason for her pain. He also knew that even if the disk had been ruptured, surgery to remove the disk would not be likely to help her pain; in fact, he believed that surgery would make her low back pain worse. He had very little to offer her, although he did give her a prescription for Lorcet®, which she said only "took the edge" off the pain.

Over the next weeks and months, and despite the fact that she spent as much time resting as she could, Nancy's pain continued to increase. She was unable to return to the job she enjoyed, and her pain made it hard to get a good night's sleep. She also was unable to participate in the sports she enjoyed so much. Her husband took over many of the household chores she used to perform so that she would not have to do activities that made her pain worse.

Because she was so inactive, she began to gain weight. She concluded that she had little control over pain or its effects on her life. She became very worried about her future, and worried that her pain was just going to get worse and worse. Eventually, she concluded that her life was ruined because of the pain.

What is happening to Nancy is understandable. But what she has concluded about her pain, and how she is now coping with it, may be making her pain worse than it has to be. In fact, even though there may not (yet) be a medical cure for back pain problems like the one that Nancy has, there *are* things that Nancy can do to get more control over her pain and her life. She *can* feel better. For this to happen, she may need to rethink the pain problem, and consider learning new ways to cope with the pain and her activity level.

How Thoughts Influence Pain

Thoughts are the words that go through your mind. Sometimes you are aware of your thoughts, like when you talk quietly to yourself.

But many times your thoughts happen automatically, and they can even occur below your awareness. You are, however, very aware of the *effects* of your thoughts. In fact, how good or bad you feel is determined in large part by the thoughts and ideas—the words—that you have in your mind at any one time.

If someone cuts you off in traffic and you think, "Hmmm, that driver must be in a hurry. Perhaps he is late for a very important appointment," you will feel much differently than if you think, "Geez! He almost caused me to have an accident! As if I didn't already have enough problems today!" More importantly, and remembering that the part of your brain that contributes to your thoughts about pain (prefrontal cortex) is directly connected to the parts of your brain that determine how unpleasant pain is (anterior cingulate cortex) and how intense the pain is (sensory cortices), we know that *the thoughts you have about pain will influence how intense the pain is and how it makes you feel.*

Helpful Thoughts and Unhelpful Thoughts

Knowing that thoughts influence how people feel, over the past 20 years, scientists have sought to discover the kinds of thoughts that are *most closely* associated with pain and its impact. The thoughts that they have identified in this research are listed in Table 2.1.

These thoughts can be classified as being helpful or unhelpful. Helpful thoughts help you feel better. They encourage you to focus less on pain and more on what is most important to you and your life. They are calming and reassuring. Anything that calms the brain will make it less responsive to painful input. On the other hand, unhelpful thoughts will make you focus more on pain and contribute to anxiety; they make your brain less calm. All by itself this is enough to increase the pain that you feel.

Using the thoughts listed in Table 2.1 as a guide, you should be able to determine whether Nancy may be hurting more than she has to, based on her thoughts about pain. Recall that she believes that she has "little control over pain or its effects on her life," that she was worried that her pain "was just going to get worse and worse," and that her "life was ruined because of the pain." These conclusions are understandable, based on the evidence available to Nancy. But, at

Table 2.1 Helpful and Unhelpful Thoughts about Pain

Helpful Thoughts

I can control my pain. I have the skills and the resources I need to influence the amount of pain I feel, and the effects that pain has on my life.

I can get on with my life. I can live a life consistent with my most deeply held values no matter what else is happening.

Unhelpful Thoughts

My pain is a catastrophe! My life has been *ruined* by pain, and I am not able to do *anything* that brings me any pleasure. It will *never* get better!

I am disabled. Because of my pain, I am not able to work or contribute to my family.

Pain is a signal of harm. Pain is a signal that physical damage is occurring. I should stop whatever I am doing when I feel pain, so that I do not injure myself further.

Some doctor, somewhere, knows of a medical cure for my pain. I should keep looking to find a doctor who will have a cure for pain, whether it be a new surgery, new medical procedure, or new medication. I should put my life on hold until I eliminate my pain.

Medications are a good way to manage pain. I will always need to take pain medications.

My family should treat me with care and concern when I hurt. Because I am fragile, especially when my pain is severe, I should be taken care of when I hurt.

---

the same time, *they are not necessarily true.* The truth is that it is possible for Nancy to get more control over pain and its effects on her life, that her pain can become less intense, and that she can engage in many activities that are important to her despite pain.

One way that Nancy can start to feel better is to replace unhelpful thoughts with more helpful and reassuring ones. This can be accomplished simply by focusing on and pondering the helpful thoughts that she believes to be true. When she learns strategies for relieving pain, she will have evidence to start to say to herself, "I have the ability to control pain and its effects on my life." As she starts to focus less on pain and more on activities that are important to her, she can say to herself, "I can live a life consistent with my most deeply held values no matter what else is happening." These are more calming and reassuring thoughts. Just focusing on such thoughts and letting them sink in will make her feel better.

An important part of learning to better manage pain, then, is to identify the pain-related beliefs that might be holding you back or making you focus more on pain than you have to. Next, you can identify the thoughts that will be more reassuring and helpful. These helpful thoughts will make it easier to feel better and meet your goals. Your clinician can also help you to identify the most helpful thoughts. Once you have a list of the helpful thoughts you think you should focus on, you can then start to use self-hypnosis strategies for increasing your mind's focus on these helpful thoughts; and feel better as a result.

Helpful and Unhelpful Thought Assessment

To help you determine the kinds of thoughts you have about your pain, you can complete the questionnaire on page 22 and then score your responses according to the instructions provided. The score can range from 0 to 32. A high score, say 28 to 32, means that you are able to avoid many of the unhelpful pain thoughts and are thinking many helpful thoughts about your pain. Good job! In this case, your thoughts are probably helping you to feel better and more reassured as you cope with pain.

A higher-than-average score, say 16 to 27, means that you are generally thinking more helpful thoughts rather than less helpful thoughts. It may be possible in this case for you to enhance your helpful thinking so that you can feel even better than you do now. You should discuss your responses to the questionnaire with your clinician and determine which thoughts, if any, you might want to focus on in treatment.

A lower-than-average score—anything less than 16—means that you have the opportunity to make some important changes in your thinking in order to be able to feel and do better. In fact, people with the lowest scores tend to show the most improvement in treatments that target pain-related thoughts; they have more room to grow! If your score on the Helpful and Unhelpful Thoughts Questionnaire is less than 16, it is strongly recommended that you work closely with your clinician to identify more reassuring and helpful thoughts that you could focus on. Bringing your responses to the questionnaire to your next session would be a first step to do this.

Helpful and Unhelpful Pain Thoughts Questionnaire

Instructions: Please circle the number that best indicates how much you believe the following thoughts about your pain, using the following scale:

0 = I do not believe this thought at all.

1 = I do not believe this thought.

2 = This thought might possibly be true.

3 = This thought is probably true.

4 = This thought is definitely true.

1. I have the skills and the resources I need to influence the amount of pain I feel, and the effects that pain has on my life...0 1 2 3 4

2. I can live a life consistent with my most deeply held values no matter what else is happening...0 1 2 3 4

3. My life has been *ruined* by pain, and I am not able to do *anything* that brings me any pleasure. It will *never* get better!...0 1 2 3 4

4. Because of my pain, I am not able to work or contribute to my family. 0 1 2 3 4

5. Pain is a signal that physical damage is occurring. I should stop whatever I am doing when I feel pain, so that I do not injure myself further. 0 1 2 3 4

6. I should put my life on hold until I eliminate my pain...0 1 2 3 4

7. I will always need to take pain medications. 0 1 2 3 4

8. When my pain is severe, I should be taken care of 0 1 2 3 4

1. First, reverse score your responses to items 3–8 by subtracting the number you circled from 4, and add them together into a single score:

   4 – Item 3 response = _____

   4 – Item 4 response = _____

   4 – Item 5 response = _____

   4 – Item 6 response = _____

   4 – Item 7 response = _____

   4 – Item 8 response = _____

   _____

   Sum = _____

2. Next, add your responses to items 1 and 2 to this number:

   Sum of reverse-scored items from above = _____

   Item 1 response = _____

   Item 2 response = _____

   _____

   Sum = _____

This sum is your total Helpful and Unhelpful Pain Thoughts Questionnaire Score. It can range from 0 to 32.

In addition to what you think about your pain, what you *do* to cope with pain will also affect how much pain you feel. One concept that many people with chronic pain do not always understand at first is that *many things we do to feel less pain in the short run can actually cause more pain in the long run.* The opposite is also often true: many of the things that we do to cope with pain that may seem difficult at first get easier with practice, and result in less pain in the long run.

The two prime examples of unhelpful coping that can produce an immediate short-term decrease in pain but a longer-term increase in pain are (1) resting and (2) using analgesic medications. You will remember that Nancy used rest as a way to minimize her pain—yet her pain problem continued to get worse. *This was because excessive rest is not good for the body, and can increase pain over time.* People with muscle pain often have chronic muscle spasms (in patients with low back pain, the spasms tend to occur deep in the back and result in "knotted" muscles that are sore when pressed) that contribute to the input that the brain is interpreting as pain. Rest does not cure chronic muscle spasms, but stretching and strengthening those muscles, as long as it is done safely and appropriately, can decrease muscle spasm in the long run. What can make this difficult for some patients is that stretching and strengthening muscles that are in spasm can result in an initial increase in pain, until the muscles get used to the exercises. This short-term increase in pain is one reason that exercise programs should often be designed and supervised by your doctor or an experienced physical therapist. You and your doctor will want to be certain that even if there is an increase in pain at first, it is *safe* to continue with the exercise program. As you increase your strength and flexibility, the spasms should decrease, as should your average pain intensity.

An unhelpful coping response that is closely related to resting is *guarding*. Guarding is a way of not using a specific body area that hurts. For example, if you feel pain in your neck, and then hold your neck very stiffly, you are guarding use of the neck. When turning your head to look at something, you might turn your torso instead of your neck. Limping is a way of guarding use of a leg. People with pain in an arm who choose to limit the use of that arm—for example, by using only or mostly the other arm—are guarding the use of the painful arm. Guarding has the same effect on the body part being guarded as resting does on the whole body. The muscles and tendons in the guarded body part tend to atrophy, making them more likely to be painful when you do try and use them.

A next step for Nancy would be to find a doctor who specializes in pain rehabilitation and have a thorough medical evaluation to make sure that it is safe to exercise, even if exercise produces more pain at first. Exercise is safe for most people with low back pain, but it is essential to have a medical evaluation to confirm this. Once the safety of exercise has been confirmed, Nancy could see a physical therapist who would help her develop a home-based exercise program that would stretch and strengthen the muscles and tendons in and around her low back.

Nancy also fell into the trap of letting her husband take over some of her chores. Like resting, avoiding chores that require physical activity can decrease pain in the short run. However, anything that restricts movement and activity has the potential to weaken muscles, and therefore make pain worse over time. Like most patients with chronic pain, Nancy will do better over time if she can avoid letting other people do things for her.

On the other hand, obtaining *emotional* support—for example, by seeking out and spending time with a loved one—can be very helpful. While this may not increase strength and flexibility like exercising and stretching can, it can make you feel less sad and hopeless, and give you something to focus on other than pain. Other helpful coping responses include (1) purposefully thinking helpful and reassuring thoughts (called *coping self-statements*), (2) maintaining an appropriate level of activity that allows you to remain strong and active, despite pain (called *pacing*), and (3) not allowing pain to interfere with your planned activities (called *task persistence*). All of the helpful coping responses listed in Table 2.2 that have been found by scientists to be associated with less pain and more activity level share a common thread: they all encourage thoughts or activities that pull attention away from pain. Many of these coping responses also help to maintain or increase strength and flexibility.

Table 2.2 Helpful and Unhelpful Coping Responses to Pain

Coping Response	Description
Helpful Coping Responses	
Coping Self-Statements	Purposefully thinking helpful and reassuring thoughts
Pacing	Maintaining an appropriate level of activity, despite pain
Task Persistence	Not allowing pain to interfere with activities
Exercise/Stretch	Engaging in muscle strengthening and stretching activity
Seeking Social Support	Finding a friend or loved one to talk to
Unhelpful Coping Responses	
Guarding	Restricting the use or movement of a body part
Resting	Engaging in a "resting" activity in response to pain, such as lying down, sitting down, or going to a dark or quiet room
Asking for Assistance	Asking someone for assistance with some activity when in pain, such as household chores or lifting

Patients who use the helpful pain coping responses *regularly* (every day or just about every day) and are able to avoid use of the unhelpful coping strategies should feel less pain and be more active than those who continue to use unhelpful strategies. But switching from unhelpful to helpful pain coping strategies can be challenging, especially at first. You should be working with your healthcare provider to get advice for and assistance with making this switch, if you both determine that it would be useful. Hypnosis can make these changes easier (see Chapter 9).

Helpful and Unhelpful Coping Assessment

To help you determine how helpful the strategies are that you are now using to cope with your pain, you can complete the Helpful and Unhelpful Pain Coping Questionnaire on page 28 and then score your responses according to the instructions provided. The score can range from 0 to 63. A very high score (in the 56-to-63 range) means that you are coping with your pain in a way that should minimize your pain and its impact on your life in the long run.

A higher-than-average score (in the 32-to-62 range) means that you are generally using more helpful coping strategies rather than less helpful ones. In this case, it should be possible for you to be able to enhance your helpful coping even further, which should make you feel better in the long run. A lower-than-average score (anything less than 32) means that you have the opportunity to make some positive changes in the way that you are coping with your pain. You should consider working with your clinician to develop a plan for engaging in helpful pain coping responses more often than you do now. You should discuss your responses to the questionnaire with your clinician and determine which adaptive coping strategies you might want to consider doing more often as your treatment progresses.

Helpful and Unhelpful Pain Coping Questionnaire

Instructions: Please circle the number of days that you used the pain coping strategies listed below in the past week, from 0 to 7 days:

On how many days in the past week did you...? Number of days ——————————

1. Purposefully think helpful and reassuring thoughts 0 1 2 3 4 5 6 7

2. Maintain a steady level of healthy activity, despite pain. 0 1 2 3 4 5 6 7

3. Not allow pain to interfere with what you planned to do..........................0 1 2 3 4 5 6 7

4. Engage in muscle-strengthening exercises 0 1 2 3 4 5 6 7

5. Engage in muscle-stretching exercises. 0 1 2 3 4 5 6 7

6. Speak with a friend or loved one for support 0 1 2 3 4 5 6 7

7. Restrict the use or movement of a body part...0 1 2 3 4 5 6 7

8. Engage in a "resting" activity in response to pain, such as lying down, sitting down, or going to a dark or quiet room...0 1 2 3 4 5 6 7

9. Ask someone for help with a household or other chore when in pain 0 1 2 3 4 5 6 7

How to Compute Your Pain Coping Score

1. First, reverse score your responses to items 7–9, by subtracting the number you circled from 4, and add them together into a single score:

    4 – Item 7 response = _____

    4 – Item 8 response = _____

    4 – Item 9 response = _____

    _____

    Sum = _____

2. Next, add your responses to items 1–6 to this number:

    Sum of reverse scored items from above = _____

    Item 1 response = _____

    Item 2 response = _____

    Item 3 response = _____

    Item 4 response = _____

    Item 5 response = _____

    Item 6 response = _____

    _____

    Sum = _____

This sum is your total Helpful and Unhelpful Pain Coping Questionnaire Score.

Copyright © Mark P. Jensen, 2011

This chapter summarized the current state-of-the-science understanding about the effects of pain-related thoughts and coping with pain. Some thoughts and coping responses will make you feel better, and you should seek to increase these. On the other hand, unhelpful beliefs and coping responses, while perhaps making you feel better in the short run, can make you feel worse over time. These should be replaced with more helpful thoughts and coping responses.

Based on what scientists have found, we have a pretty good picture of what a person who is managing well with chronic pain looks like. Such an individual would rarely, if ever, think alarming and unhelpful thoughts about or in response to pain. He or she would also rarely, if ever, rest in response to pain. When experiencing pain, he or she would probably not ask for help with a chore that he or she is capable of doing. Rather, this person would be thinking realistic, reassuring, and adaptive thoughts—thoughts reflecting a sense of control over pain and its effects—and would use adaptive and helpful pain coping responses to manage pain.

The helpful and unhelpful pain thoughts and pain coping questionnaires that you completed in this chapter can give you an initial idea regarding where you stand with respect to your own pain-related thoughts and coping responses. Because you can use self-hypnosis to increase your helpful thoughts and use of helpful coping, you should discuss your responses to the questionnaires you completed with your clinician. You can then decide together which of these you most want to change as a part of your hypnosis treatment.

Part II: Understanding Hypnosis

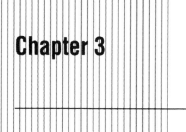

Chapter 3   *What Is Hypnosis?*

Goals

- To learn the different definitions of hypnosis

- To learn about the history of hypnosis

- To review theories of hypnosis

Chapter Overview

The history of hypnosis has not been without controversy. Even today, scientists and clinicians do not always agree on the best way(s) to define or explain the effects of hypnosis. But even if there is disagreement about *why* hypnosis works, there is not a disagreement about its efficacy: *scientists have demonstrated that hypnosis treatment effectively changes thoughts, perceptions (including pain perception), and behavior.*

This chapter provides a basic introduction to hypnosis. It discusses what hypnosis is, and the distinction between *hypnosis* and *self-hypnosis*. It then provides a summary of the history of hypnosis. The chapter ends with a review of the theories that are used to understand hypnosis and its effects.

Definition of Hypnosis

At its most basic, hypnosis can be defined as a *procedure* in which "one person (the subject) is guided by another person (the hypnotist) to respond to suggestions for changes in subjective experience, alterations in perception, sensation, emotion, thought or behavior." Hypnosis usually begins with an induction that invites the subject to focus his or her attention on a single object, sensation, or image.

This is followed by one or more suggestions for making positive changes.

Hypnosis can also be thought of in terms of its *effects*. A group of individuals may be given a hypnotic induction or hypnotic treatment, but not all of them will respond the same way. When used for pain management, some people will find that pain mostly disappears during hypnosis, while others will notice more modest effects. Some people may notice that hypnosis has a bigger effect on *how bothered they are* by their pain than on *how intense the pain feels*. It is not possible to predict ahead of time what benefits a patient will experience during and after hypnosis treatment, although nearly everyone who learns self-hypnosis reports at least some benefit, and many people report substantial benefits.

Hypnosis can also be differentiated from *self-hypnosis*. *Hypnosis* usually refers to an interaction between two people: a clinician and a patient. During hypnosis, the clinician offers hypnotic inductions and suggestions to the patient, who listens and responds. In this interaction, the goal of hypnosis treatment is not only to help the patient feel better during the session, but also to help the patient make long-lasting changes in what he or she thinks about pain, and in how his or her brain processes pain information—in other words, to extend the good feelings that occur during hypnosis sessions into the patient's day-to-day life.

Self-hypnosis refers to someone using his or her ability to experience a hypnotic trance and to feel the benefits on his or her own, outside of the clinician's office. Patients usually learn self-hypnosis in the context of hypnotic treatment, as they work with a specialist to indentify the most effective ways to experience a trance state. Once they learn self-hypnosis, they can use it many times during the day to calm the brain and to achieve specific goals—for example, to feel less pain, to make it easier to exercise, to sleep better, or simply to feel more calm and confident.

If you are working with an experienced clinician, the chances are good that he or she will be making audio recordings of your hypnosis sessions so that you can continue to use *hypnosis* between sessions and after treatment is over by simply listening to the recordings. The clinician can also teach you *self-hypnosis* by suggesting a cue you can use (for example, to take a deep breath, hold it, and then let it go) to enter a hypnotic state on your own without an audio recording. Using this cue, you can experience the hypnotic state more easily.

A Brief History of Hypnosis

It is possible to find descriptions of people using hypnosis to treat medical conditions throughout history. The ancient Egyptians had "dream temples" and the ancient Greeks had "sleep temples" where hypnotic suggestions were used to help treat symptoms. Most historians agree, however, that the origins of the modern scientific examination of hypnosis began with Anton Mesmer (1734–1815). Mesmer was a physician practicing in Paris in the late 1700s. He believed that bodily tissues held magnetic energy, and that this energy could be directed, using magnets, to ease symptoms and heal disease. He also believed that some people had more magnetic energy (*animal magnetism*) than others. These people could be very effective healers if they focused and directed this energy.

Mesmer's treatment involved having patients sit around a *baquet* (a tub filled with water and iron fillings) and hold on to iron rods that stuck out of the baquet. He would then seek to guide healing magnetic energy through the patients. When treated in this way, his patients would go into convulsions and be taken to a recovery room. As they recovered from the experience, many reported being "cured" of their disease or symptoms.

Mesmer's treatments were so effective and he became so popular that he attracted the attention of the authorities. King Louis XVI appointed a commission (which included Benjamin Franklin, who was living in Paris at the time) to study Mesmer's practice and theory of animal magnetism. The commission determined, through careful experimentation, that Mesmer's theory was incorrect. His profound results, they concluded, were "only" due to the engagement of the imagination of his patients.

The commission recommended that the potential beneficial effects of engaging a patient's imagination to relieve symptoms be studied further. However, this advice was not followed at the time. In fact, it took another 200 years before serious research into the effects and efficacy of hypnotic suggestions started. When the commission dismissed Mesmer's theory of animal magnetism, Mesmer himself was discredited. He left Paris, and his disgrace made many in the mainstream hesitant to use or study mesmerism. As a result, interest in mesmerism plummeted over the next few decades.

In the mid-1800s, books about mesmerism were translated into English and published in the United Kingdom and United States. An English surgeon working in Calcutta, India, used it as an anesthetic for surgery at this time and reported very positive outcomes. Both of these things brought back an interest in mesmerism. However, just as the positive findings about hypnosis as a surgical anesthetic were published, both chloroform and ether were discovered and found to be so effective that interest in mesmerism for this purpose never caught on. Mesmerism came to be called *hypnosis* (a term coined by an English physician in the 1840s) to separate it from the negative history associated with Mesmer's (discredited) idea that its effects were associated with magnetic currents.

In the 1870s, interest in hypnosis revived, in large part due to a number of prominent French neurologists, including Jean-Martin Charcot (1825–1893) and Hippolyte Bernheim (1840–1919), who became interested in its effects. Charcot believed that hypnosis could be used to induce and then study various neurological conditions. His prominence and respect gave back much of the credibility the study of hypnosis had lost during Mesmer's time.

Bernheim was particularly interested in the clinical benefits of hypnosis. With Ambroise-Auguste Liébeault (1823–1904), another prominent clinician, he founded the "Nancy School" of hypnosis to further promote its therapeutic role. Pierre Janet (1859–1947), a psychologist and student of both Charcot's and Bernheim's, had an active hypnosis practice in Paris. Janet's published work includes some of the first case reports of the effective clinical use of hypnosis for conditions such as anorexia nervosa.

In the late 1880s, Sigmund Freud (1856–1939) visited Charcot and Bernheim in Paris to learn more about hypnosis and its clinical application. He began using hypnosis in his practice, and through its use developed his theory of the unconscious mind. However, he later replaced hypnosis with other procedures he developed himself, such as dream analysis. The specific reasons for his loss of interest in hypnosis are not clear, although some argue that the high degree of rapport required for effective hypnotic practice may have been inconsistent with Freud's personality and preferred clinical approach. In any case, Freud's abandonment of hypnosis, combined with the rise in acceptance of psychoanalysis, has been blamed as a primary cause of the decline of interest in hypnosis in the early 1900s.

In the 1930s, the published works of two individuals, one a prominent psychologist and researcher and the other a prominent psychiatrist, brought a resurgence of interest in hypnosis. First, Clark Hull (1884–1952), a highly respected experimental psychologist, published a book in 1933 that presented the results of highly controlled experiments using hypnosis. Hull's findings regarding the effects of hypnosis on a person's ability to alter pain gave hypnosis a high degree of scientific credibility. Second, Milton H. Erickson (1902–1980), a practicing psychiatrist, began publishing the results of his creative use of hypnosis and hypnotic language to help his patients manage a variety of symptoms and problems.

Ernest R. Hilgard (1904–2001), a professor of psychology at Stanford University, designed and completed many groundbreaking laboratory experiments on the effects of hypnosis and hypnotic analgesia. His work, published in some of the most prominent and well-respected scientific journals, built on that of Hull's and gave hypnosis even more scientific credibility. Hilgard also developed a theoretical model of hypnosis that remains one of the prominent theories today. Much of the scientific psychological research in the field during this period, and into the late 1900s, focused on developing, testing, and comparing different theories of hypnosis. At times, the debates regarding these models became quite contentious, and echoes of this controversy remain today.

The first decade of the 21st century saw a dramatic increase in scientific research on hypnosis, especially on the use of hypnosis for pain management. Much of this research focused on how hypnosis alters brain activity, as well as its clinical efficacy. The key findings from this research are summarized in the next chapter.

This section of the chapter describes three different theories on how hypnosis works. One theory describes the effects of hypnosis from the perspective of the psychology of the mind, one from the perspective of social interactions, and one from the perspective of the biology of the brain. Together, these theories can help us to better understand that the apparent "magic" of hypnosis is not magic at all. Response to hypnosis is as natural and real as any of the many other amazing things human beings can learn to do, such as reading, speaking, or playing a musical instrument.

The Psychology of the Mind: Dissociation Theories of Hypnosis

Earnest Hilgard, the Stanford researcher mentioned earlier who nurtured scientific interest in hypnosis starting in the 1950s, was lecturing to a large class on hypnosis, demonstrating the concept of hypnotically induced deafness. After a hypnotic suggestion for deafness, the student he had hypnotized in front of the class seemed unable to hear anything, including a loud clap of the hands. One of the students in the class asked if a *part* of the student who appeared to be deaf could still hear at some level. Hilgard found this to be a very interesting question, and simply asked the student this question while the student was still under hypnosis. The student's response was that a part of him could hear the noises in the room, but not the part that was currently in communication with Dr. Hilgard. This example is a good illustration of the concept of *dissociation*—that certain parts of consciousness can split off from one another—as an explanation for what happens with hypnosis.

Pierre Janet was the first to hypothesize that dissociation was at the core of hypnosis. Based on the experience just described and others like it, Ernest Hilgard developed a theory of hypnosis that he termed the *neo*dissociation model to distinguish it from Janet's approach. Hilgard's theory asserts that the human mind is organized into subunits, and that all of these subunits are usually under the control of an *executive ego*. The executive ego is responsible for monitoring the entire system and initiating action.

When the patient was hypnotized, and following an appropriate suggestion, Hilgard thought that the executive ego "let go" of some of its control over the mind. This allows the parts of the brain that usually work together in concert to work separately. It makes it possible, for example, for the parts of the brain that process pain sensations to disconnect from the part of the brain that gives us an awareness of sensory information. The brain may still be processing pain, but we no longer feel the pain. Imagine, for example, if all forms of communication were cut between Los Angeles, St. Louis, and New York. People living in each of these towns could not know what was happening in the other towns. If the people in the New York office were responsible for determining how much pain you had, the people in the St. Louis office were responsible for determining how upset you are about pain, and you were in the "head office" in Los Angeles, you would not be aware of any pain or suffering associated with pain. You could feel fine, even if the people in New York and St. Louis are complaining. Hilgard thought that dissociation was one of the brain's natural responses to focusing one's attention, as occurs with hypnosis.

Social Interactions: Sociocognitive Views of Hypnosis

The "*socio*" in *sociocognitive* stands for the parts of the theory that relate to social contexts, and the "*cognitive*" piece stands for the parts of the theory that relate to thoughts or beliefs. Sociocognitive theorists note that people tend to do what they think is expected of them in social situations. In this view, hypnotic interactions are not different from any other social interaction. Sociocognitivists believe that people respond to hypnosis and hypnotic suggestions because they think that they should and because they want to. In other words, with hypnosis, no one is forcing anyone to do anything he or she does not really want to do. Response to hypnosis is voluntary.

Brain Biology: Neurophysiologic Views of Hypnosis

A number of scientists have studied hypnosis from the perspective of *neurophysiology* (*neuro* for nerve and *physiology* for the biological functions of those nerves) or brain activity. Neurophysiologists have discovered that the brain activity in people who respond to hypnosis is different than the brain activity in people who do not respond to hypnosis. In other words, hypnosis has measurable effects on the brain. Interestingly, brain areas influenced by hypnosis—including the front of the brain (e.g., prefrontal cortex) and the anterior cingulate cortex (ACC)—are also brain areas involved in the processing of pain. This research has also shown that overall electrical activity in the brain decreases when people are hypnotized; hypnosis calms the brain. When the brain is calmer, it processes less information, including less information about pain. Thus, hypnosis can be seen as a way to teach people to control their overall brain activity and brain activity in specific areas. Both of these help people to feel more comfortable.

Chapter Summary

Hypnosis has a very long history, and its popularity has waxed and waned over the years. However, throughout its history, clinicians have noted that hypnosis can effectively help people with medical problems; in particular, it can help people to feel less pain. Different theories have been proposed to explain the effects of hypnosis, and each theory helps us to understand a little more about how hypnosis works. Dissociation theories provide a useful understanding for how our mind can separate into parts to decrease the amount of pain we feel during and after hypnotic analgesia suggestions. Sociocognitive models emphasize the importance of the social and personal interaction between the clinician and the subject, as well as the role of motivation and expectations. Neurophysiologic models provide a description of the biological underpinnings of hypnosis. All of these theories help us to understand that there is nothing "magical" or mysterious about hypnosis. Its effects and benefits are very real.

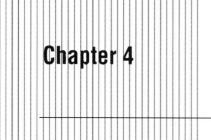

Chapter 4   *What Hypnosis Can Do for Pain*

Goals

- To understand the effects of hypnosis on the brain areas that create our experience of pain

- To learn about the effects of hypnosis and self-hypnosis training on chronic pain

- To understand how you might use this knowledge to benefit from hypnosis and self-hypnosis

Chapter Overview

Many scientists have studied the effects of hypnosis on pain. Their research can be divided into two general areas: (1) laboratory studies looking at the biological effects of hypnosis on the parts of the brain responsible for creating the experience of pain and (2) clinical studies measuring levels of chronic pain before and after hypnosis treatment and self-hypnosis training. This chapter describes the findings from both types of research, and discusses what these findings mean for helping you to benefit from hypnosis.

Effects of Hypnosis on Activity in Brain Areas that Create the Experience of Pain

Chapter 1 of this workbook reviewed what we now know about how the body and brain work together to create the experience of pain. One of the most important conclusions from this knowledge is the understanding that the brain is *not* merely a passive recipient of the information it receives from sensors in the skin, muscles, and bones. Rather, the brain actively processes the information it receives to create everything that we experience, including our sense of pain and how much pain bothers us. Depending on many factors, the brain may create more or less pain. Hypnosis can alter how the brain processes pain information, which means that you can learn to use hypnosis to hurt less. You will remember from Chapter 1 that activity in pain sensors in the periphery (the area of the body outside of the spinal cord and brain) and activity in the spine and in certain areas of the brain all contribute to the experience of pain. As it turns out, hypnosis influences activity in *all* of these areas.

Effects of Hypnosis on the Periphery

Research shows that hypnosis influences the levels of chemicals in the skin that make pain sensors more or less sensitive to noxious stimulation. In one study, for example, researchers compared responses to noxious heat administered to the right and left arms of subjects following hypnotic suggestions for one arm to be "normal" and the other arm to be "vulnerable." Following the hypnotic suggestions, both arms were exposed to high levels of heat. The investigators found more inflammatory reactions and tissue damage in the skin of the "vulnerable" than the "normal" arms. They then compared responses to hypnotic suggestions that one arm would be "anesthetic" (have no sensations) and the other arm would be "vulnerable." In this second study, they found greater inflammatory reactions and tissue damage in the "vulnerable" arm relative to the "anesthetic" arm. They also found a greater increase in a chemical in the arm that makes the sensors in the skin more sensitive to pain in the "vulnerable" arm than the "anesthetic" arm. Thus, if the pain that you feel is due, at least in part, to the stimulation of pain sensors in the periphery (your skin, muscles, or bones), you could potentially learn to use hypnosis to reduce the sensitivity of those sensors so that you feel less pain.

Effects of Hypnosis on Nerves in the Spine

There is also evidence that hypnosis can influence nervous system activity in the spinal cord and decrease the pain information that is allowed into the spinal cord. Research in this area has studied the effects on spinal *reflexes*. A reflex is an involuntary (and nearly instantaneous) response to a stimulus. Reflex responses are not initiated by the brain; they are initiated by nerves in the spinal cord. This allows reflex actions to occur very quickly, which can help us to protect our arms and legs from physical damage when the pain sensors start to detect the potential for damage. A reflex is the reason your hand will automatically pull away from a source of heat even before you become aware of any heat.

The reflex response that most people are aware of is the *patellar reflex*. Doctors test this reflex by tapping the patellar tendon (the tendon just below the knee). In a person with an intact nervous system, the tap will send a message to the spine, which then sends a message immediately back to the muscles in the leg to extend the lower leg, producing an automatic "kick." Scientists have found that when given hypnotic suggestions for decreased pain in response to noxious stimulation, subjects show changes in spinal reflexes. This provides direct evidence that hypnosis influences activity in the spine. It also means that you may be able to learn to use hypnosis to alter pain by altering how much painful input nerves in the spine let in.

Effects of Hypnosis on Brain Activity

In the past decade, there have been significant advances in our ability to view and measure activity in the brain with fMRI, EEG, and PET scans. Scientists studying hypnosis have taken advantage of these advances to determine whether (and where) hypnosis affects brain activity. One important finding from this research is that hypnosis can be very precise in targeting activity in specific areas of the brain. For example, hypnotic suggestions for decreased pain *unpleasantness* have been shown to produce decreased activity in the anterior cingulate cortex (ACC), but not the sensory cortices. Recall from Chapter 1 that the ACC is involved with processing the emotional (suffering), but not the sensory (intensity), aspects of pain. In a follow-up study, these same scientists found that hypnotic suggestions for decreased pain *intensity* produced decreased activity in the sensory cortex but not the ACC.

In another study, researchers measured brain activity under three different experimental conditions: (1) during noxious heat stimulation, (2) after hypnotic suggestions that the subjects will experience the same pain they felt during the noxious heat stimulation (but without the painful stimulation present), and (3) after a request that the subjects simply think about or imagine the pain. The average pain intensity rating (on 0–10 scales) during actual noxious stimulation was 5.7, and the average pain rating following hypnotic suggestions to re-experience this pain was 2.8. None of the subjects in this study reported that they experienced pain during the "imagined" pain condition. Interestingly, the same brain areas active following noxious stimulation were also active following hypnotic suggestions for pain, including the thalamus, ACC, insula, and prefrontal cortex. This research is striking in that it shows that hypnotic suggestions without physical stimulation can create pain sensations, and that the brain behaves similarly when it feels "hypnotic pain" to how it behaves in response to noxious input. In both cases, of course, the pain is real, because it is the brain that creates pain. Also, if the brain can create the sensation of pain with hypnosis, the brain should be able to create the sensation of comfort and relaxation with hypnosis. In short, hypnosis has clear and measurable biological effects on activity in the areas of the brain that create the experience of pain.

What Knowledge about the Effects of Hypnosis on Brain Activity Means for You

In the past, clinicians who used hypnosis to help people with chronic pain tended to give just one or two hypnotic suggestions for pain relief. They also mostly targeted only the sensory components of pain (for example, they might suggest a decrease in pain intensity). But we now know that hypnosis can affect activity in *all* of the areas of the brain and body that influence pain, not just areas involved in the processing of the sensory aspects of pain. Hypnosis can also decrease (1) activity at the site of any ongoing physical damage or inflammatory responses in the periphery, (2) how much pain information is allowed into the spinal cord, (3) activity in the ACC that affects how much the pain bothers you, (4) activity in the sensory cortices that affects how intense the pain feels to you, (5) activity in the prefrontal cortex that influences the thoughts you have about pain, and (6) activity in the insula that affects whether you feel obliged to do anything to cope with or reduce pain.

Chapter 7 of this workbook and the treatment protocol in the accompanying therapist guide both include hypnotic suggestions that affect all of these components of pain. Your job will be to keep track of which hypnotic suggestions work the best for you, and use this information to design, with your therapist, the most effective hypnotic protocol for your unique pain problem.

Effects of Hypnotic Treatments on Chronic Pain

In the past two decades, and in particular in the past ten years, a number of well-controlled research studies have investigated the efficacy of self-hypnosis for chronic pain management. The results from these studies are consistent: when compared to standard care, hypnosis is effective for reducing chronic daily pain, and the beneficial effects of hypnosis tend to last for as long as follow-up data are collected—up to one year in some studies. If the benefits last this long, there is no reason to expect that they would not last even longer. Hypnosis has also been found to be either as effective or more effective than other treatments for reducing chronic pain, including medications and physical therapy. As a group, the research results provide strong evidence for the efficacy of hypnosis, and reinforce the importance of considering this as a treatment option for patients who are interested in learning this treatment approach.

This section provides some specific details from a number of research studies that make the following five additional important points: (1) response to hypnosis treatment varies from person to person; (2) you need not be "highly hypnotizable" to benefit from hypnotic treatment; (3) the "side effects" of hypnosis treatment are overwhelmingly positive; (4) you can reasonably expect two types of positive outcomes following hypnosis treatment for pain: a reduction in the severity of ongoing daily pain, and an ability to use self-hypnosis to experience periods of comfort; and (5) patients and clinicians should consider using hypnosis to alter *more* than just pain intensity.

Response to Hypnosis Treatment Varies from Person to Person

In 2005 a group of us studied the short- and long-term effects of 10 sessions of self-hypnosis training in 33 individuals with chronic pain associated with various physical disabilities (spinal cord injury, multiple sclerosis, and acquired amputation, among others). We followed this study with two additional clinical trials comparing the effects of the hypnotic treatment protocol with two other viable treatments: biofeedback and relaxation training.

In all three studies, almost all (about 80%) of the patients reported immediate and substantial reductions in pain *when they were hypnotized*. When the hypnosis session ended, most of the patients who felt immediate pain relief during the hypnosis sessions reported that the pain reduction they felt with hypnosis lasted for several hours (and sometimes for days or even longer).

In terms of average daily pain—the pain that the patients in these studies reported feeling in their day-to-day lives before and after treatment—hypnosis was found to result in significant pain decreases in many patients. Follow-up studies showed that when treatment produced a reduction in pain, that reduction lasted for at least 12 months. However, not *everyone* who received the treatment reported large decreases in daily pain. Based on these research findings, it is not reasonable to expect hypnosis to produce a miraculous cure in everyone who tries it. However, it is also not reasonable to conclude that hypnosis and self-hypnosis training cannot help. The findings clearly show us that *hypnosis treatment helps many people*. Moreover, when it helps, its benefits are shown to last for at least 12 months, and maybe longer.

You Need Not be "Highly Hypnotizable" to Benefit from Hypnosis Treatment

Hypnotizability is a person's ability to respond to a large variety of hypnotic suggestions. Hypnotizability can be viewed as a trait or talent, much like intelligence or musical ability. It has also been shown highly stable across time—as stable over the years and decades, in fact, as IQ test scores.

Given its strong stability over time, some clinicians think that it is useful to measure hypnotizability and then use the resulting hypnotizability score to screen patients into (this would be those who score high) or out of (this would be those who score low) hypnotic treatment. However, research has shown that general hypnotizability is associated with only *some* measures of treatment outcome in *some* studies. Moreover, when relationships are found between hypnotizability scores and treatment outcome, they tend to be weak. Overall, the scientific evidence indicates that *hypnotizability plays, at most, a small role in the outcome of hypnotic treatment of chronic pain.* Therefore, many individuals who score low on measures of hypnotizability can still benefit from hypnotic treatments, and measures of hypnotizability should *not* be used to screen patients into or out of hypnotic treatment. If the clinician you are working with administers a hypnotizability test, it is likely that he or she is only trying to identify how you are responding to different types of hypnotic inductions and suggestions, in order to design a hypnosis treatment program that fits with how you respond. He or she should not be using the test to screen you out of treatment.

The "Side Effects" of Hypnosis Treatment are Overwhelmingly Positive

The clinicians who provided treatment in the studies we have completed noted nearly universal patient satisfaction with hypnosis treatment. To better understand the reasons for such a high satisfaction rate, we performed a follow-up study, asking the participants to describe all of the benefits they obtained with the hypnosis treatment.

Only one (3%) of the participants contacted reported no benefits. *That means that 97% of the participants reported at least some benefit from this treatment!* The treatment benefits that were mentioned were classified into pain-related, non-pain-related, or neutral benefits. Forty unique types of benefits were described by the participants, and only nine (23%) of these were related to pain. The most common pain-related benefits listed by the participants were (1) pain reduction, (2) increased sense of control over pain, and (3) a sense of having a new option or tool to deal with pain. Many more of the benefits from the treatment were non-pain-related; they included (1) an increase in positive mood, relaxation, and sense of well-being, (2) increased energy, (3) increased self-awareness, and (4) lowered blood pressure. In short, even though the specific focus of the hypnotic treatment was to decrease pain intensity, the individuals who received self-hypnosis training reported a large number of additional benefits, which contributed to their being highly satisfied with hypnosis treatment.

Thus, as you participate in treatment, you can expect to notice some benefits over and above those associated with your pain. You may find that you are sleeping better, feel more energy, and have an increased sense of well-being throughout the day. It would be a good idea to note these additional benefits when they occur, and report them to your therapist. Together, you may decide to build on them by including hypnotic suggestions in future sessions that these benefits will occur again (and even, if appropriate, become permanent).

Hypnosis Has at Least Two Types of Outcome on Pain Intensity

To understand the effects of self-hypnosis training after treatment, we contacted the participants in the study at different time points. We wanted to learn how often the patients listened to the audio recordings of the treatment sessions and how often they practiced the self-hypnosis skills they were taught. We also asked them to rate the amount of pain relief they had when they listened to the recordings or practiced self-hypnosis, and how long that pain relief lasted.

We learned that three months after treatment, up to 85% of the participants who received self-hypnosis training still listened to the audio recordings of sessions (on audio tapes or CDs that were given to them), and up to 80% continued to practice self-hypnosis on their own without an audio recording. The people who listened to the recordings or practiced self-hypnosis reported that they felt pain relief when they did so. The pain relief they felt tended to last for 3 to 6 hours after listening to the recordings, and 1 to 3 hours when they practiced on their own without the recordings. The fact that participants reported experiencing *immediate* reductions in pain intensity when they listened to the recordings or practiced self-hypnosis, and that fact that these reductions lasted for hours after hypnosis practice, could explain the high rates of continued use of self-hypnosis after treatment. People continue to do the things that they find useful.

As we thought about the findings from our studies, we determined that hypnosis treatment for chronic pain has two potential effects. First, it appears to produce a significant reduction in daily pain that lasts for at least 12 months (and possibly longer) after treatment in *some* (but not all) patients who receive this treatment. Second, for an even larger number of individuals—up to 85%—the treatment provides patients with audio recordings and a skill (self-hypnosis) for producing short-term reductions in pain intensity that they can experience when they choose to use either one. This latter finding, in particular, may explain the almost universal satisfaction with hypnosis treatment.

Using Hypnosis to Alter *More* than Just Pain Severity

We recently completed a study that tested the effects of expanding hypnotic suggestions to help patients decrease unhelpful pain-related thoughts, in addition to pain intensity. Our reason for performing this study was based on evidence that adding hypnosis to other treatments, such as cognitive therapy, can enhance their efficacy. We wanted to determine whether hypnotic cognitive therapy designed to reduce unhelpful pain-related thoughts and increase helpful ones could contribute to changes in pain or in the frequency of alarming cognitions.

To address this research question, we performed a study in which 15 people with chronic pain were given 16 treatment sessions: (1) four educational sessions where they were given information about pain that was designed to be useful, but was not expected to have a direct effect on either pain intensity or unhelpful thoughts; (2) four sessions of pain-focused self-hypnosis training that we thought would directly reduce pain intensity; (3) four sessions of cognition-focused cognitive therapy that we thought would directly reduce the frequency of unhelpful thoughts; and (4) four sessions of hypnotic cognitive therapy. We thought that this final treatment had the potential to reduce *both* unhelpful thoughts and pain intensity, but because it had never been tested before, we did not know how beneficial it would be. Pain intensity was assessed before and after each of the 16 individual sessions, and daily average pain intensity, worst pain intensity, frequency of unhelpful thoughts, and pain interference (the extent to which pain interfered with different activities of daily living, such as household chores and sleep) were all assessed before treatment and after each of the four treatment modules.

The results of the study were mostly as we expected, although there were some interesting surprises. First, as expected, both of the treatments that included hypnosis resulted in significant immediate (pre- to post-session) and substantial decreases in pain intensity, while the education and cognitive therapy sessions showed no such effects. These findings confirm that hypnosis results in immediate reductions in pain for most people. Second, as expected, the study participants reported significantly lower levels of average daily pain intensity, relative to the education condition, following the hypnosis treatment, but not after cognitive therapy. This finding confirmed the beneficial effects of self-hypnosis training on average daily pain.

Interestingly, however, and inconsistent with what we expected, *both* the hypnosis and the cognitive therapy conditions resulted in decreases in the frequency of unhelpful negative thoughts. We had originally thought that the cognitive therapy treatment would show greater effects for decreasing the frequency of unhelpful thoughts than the hypnosis treatment would, because cognitive therapy targets these thoughts, while the hypnosis treatment we used in the study targeted only pain intensity. This finding suggested to us that hypnosis may be useful for decreasing negative thoughts as well as pain intensity, perhaps by giving patients an increased sense of control over pain and allowing them to feel less helpless about it.

The most interesting results from this study, perhaps, were related to the combined hypnotic cognitive therapy treatment. Following the hypnotic cognitive therapy sessions, the participants reported significant improvements in everything we measured, over and above the effects of hypnosis or cognitive therapy alone. These findings suggest that pain-related cognitive therapy might be enhanced by hypnosis. For this reason, and if your therapist is using the therapist guide associated with this patient workbook, he or she will likely speak with you about using hypnosis to help you focus on helpful and reassuring thoughts.

Chapter Summary

Research, especially research performed in the past decade, has demonstrated that hypnosis has measurable effects on all of the nervous system areas that are involved in the creation of pain. Hypnosis can reduce inflammatory responses in the periphery (skin), change the modulation of input at the level of the spinal cord, and alter activity in all of the brain areas involved in the creation of pain sensations.

These research results provide clear evidence that the effects of hypnosis on pain are real. Hypnosis changes more than just a patient's willingness to report pain. It alters brain activity that underlies the experience of pain. The research results also provide a rationale for expanding hypnotic suggestions to include more than merely reductions in pain intensity.

Scientists who study the effects of hypnosis on chronic pain have found that the majority of patients who receive hypnosis will report significant and meaningful reductions in pain intensity during individual hypnosis sessions. Many of these patients will be pleasantly surprised by the effects of hypnosis, and many will be able to go on to use the audio recordings from the hypnosis treatment sessions to replicate this benefit outside of the clinic. Some patients will also achieve marked reductions in their daily pain, and these improvements last for weeks, months, and possibly indefinitely after treatment. Finally, the results of a recently completed study suggest that hypnosis may be very helpful for helping patients to decrease the frequency of unhelpful pain-related thoughts, thereby reducing the pain and suffering associated with chronic pain even further.

Part III: Using Self-Hypnosis for Chronic Pain Management

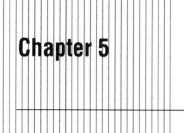

Chapter 5

Hypnosis and Self-Hypnosis for Chronic Pain Management: The Basics

Goals

- To clarify any misconceptions you may have about hypnosis

- To review what a typical hypnosis and self-hypnosis session is like

- To understand what you should be prepared to tell your clinician during your initial evaluation

Chapter Overview

The primary purpose of this chapter is to give you practical information about hypnosis as you consider participating in hypnosis treatment and incorporating self-hypnosis into your life. It begins by discussing some of the more common misconceptions that people have about hypnosis, and provides you with accurate information to address these misunderstandings. It then describes the typical structure of hypnosis sessions (the sessions you will have with your clinician) and self-hypnosis (when you use hypnosis on your own, usually at home) and how these fit into your treatment program. Finally, it reviews the important information you should be prepared to discuss with your clinician during your initial evaluation. After reading this chapter, you will be prepared to get the most out of your hypnosis treatment.

Hypnosis Myths and Misconceptions

Many people learn about hypnosis from movies and television, or from watching stage hypnotists perform. Unfortunately, almost all of what they learn from these sources is wrong. Worse, this misinformation can raise concerns or fears about hypnosis that might make you hesitant to try it. This section of the chapter provides a discussion of the myths and misconceptions that some people may have about hypnosis. It is written to reassure you that the hypnotic state is a natural response that most people already enter on a daily basis. Importantly, because the state of focused awareness that follows hypnosis is associated with greater flexibility, you can learn to use the hypnotic state to get more control over your sensations, thoughts, and feelings.

Myth: Hypnosis is the Same as Sleep

When hypnosis is portrayed in movies or television, the hypnotist sometimes induces a hypnotic response by telling the subject that he or she is getting "sleepy." Often, the hypnotic subject then closes his or her eyes and seems to enter a zombie-like state. Because of this portrayal, some people believe that hypnosis is a form of sleep, and that the subject becomes unconscious during hypnotic procedures. If you believe this, you may not think that you are receiving "real" hypnosis if you are not invited to get "sleepy." You may also believe that you will not respond well to hypnosis treatment if you do not "fall asleep" during the induction or hypnotic procedures.

Scientists have determined, however, that hypnosis is *not* the same as sleep. During sleep people are not conscious, and the brain shows a specific pattern of brain activity. No such brain activity is seen during hypnosis. In fact, *the brain activity seen during hypnosis is very similar to the brain activity observed when people feel very relaxed and focused, but are still awake.* Rather than "sleep," hypnosis can be described as a state of focused attention during which you can get more and better control of your thoughts and sensations. It is true, though, that with hypnosis there is a general calming of brain activity. For this reason, you may find that it is easier to drift off into sleep whenever you wish, once you learn self-hypnosis (see Chapter 9).

Myth: During Hypnosis the Clinician has Control over the Subject

Almost always, when hypnosis is shown in movies or on television, it involves one person (who often has evil intentions) using hypnosis to gain control over another. Sometimes the hypnotist uses hypnosis to force the hypnotic subject to do something that he or she would not otherwise consider doing. Also, stage hypnotists often use hypnosis to encourage volunteer audience members to engage in behaviors that might usually be embarrassing for them ("bark like a dog"). Some patients are worried that when they are hypnotized they might disclose, or be forced to disclose, an important secret.

However, people cannot be *forced* to do something under hypnosis they would not normally do. Self-hypnosis training is designed to give you skills to promote comfort—to give you *more* control over what you think and how you feel. Clinicians who are expert at using hypnosis do not seek to control or brainwash you. In fact, when giving suggestions, you may hear the clinician qualify the hypnotic suggestions by saying, "you will find that it is easy to respond to suggestions that are *appropriate for your comfort and well-being*." By using this wording, your clinician will be giving your mind permission to only respond to those suggestions that you think will be most helpful to you; you will be free to simply ignore the rest.

Myth: Only Weak-Minded, "Suggestible," or Gullible People Can Be Hypnotized

It is generally known that people vary in their responsivity to hypnotic suggestions. However, despite significant efforts to identify the predictors of hypnotic responsivity, researchers have not been able to identify personality traits or other individual factors that predict who will and who will not respond to hypnosis. Responding to hypnosis depends much more on your ability to use your mind and imagination than on your personality type. Luckily, the ability to use hypnosis for pain management is among the easiest of hypnotic tasks. This may explain why hypnosis is used so often for pain management, and why so many people with chronic pain seem to benefit from learning self-hypnosis skills.

Myth: You Will Lose All Conscious Awareness during Hypnosis and Have No Memory of the Experience

During hypnosis, you will probably experience something very much like what you experience on a daily basis when you are deeply absorbed in a hobby or other relaxing activity. You will likely find the hypnotic state to be pleasant, and remember most if not all of what transpired during the hypnosis sessions. Some people worry that they "did not feel hypnotized" during the procedures, because the state of hypnosis is a natural relaxed state that seems so familiar. But if you are able to feel even a little bit more relaxed during your hypnosis sessions and are able to focus your attention on the clinician's voice, or focus on your own inner experience during self-hypnosis, you will be "hypnotized" enough to benefit.

Myth: You Must Remember Everything that the Clinician Says in Order for the Session to be Effective

On the opposite end of the continuum, some people believe that they must consciously remember and process everything that is said during the hypnotic session in order to benefit from hypnosis. However, with hypnosis, people do not need to "work at" listening to everything that the clinician says. Like learning other skills, learning how to use hypnosis for pain management does not require 100% of your conscious attention at all times. You may find that you drift in and out of being aware of the clinician's voice during the sessions. If this occurs, it should have little effect, one way or the other, on how much benefit you obtain from the treatment.

Myth: If You Do Not Experience a Deep Level of Focused Attention, the Treatment Will Not Be Effective

Many people believe that the benefits of hypnosis are maximized when patients attain "deep" levels of focused attention, as opposed to "light" levels. However, there is no evidence that supports this assumption. As mentioned previously, learning to get control over and decrease pain is one of the easier hypnotic skills—possibly because we already have the nervous system wiring to make this control possible.

Myth: What Happens with Clinical Hypnosis is the Same as What Happens with Stage Hypnosis

Stage hypnosis is not the same as clinical hypnosis. First of all, the goals are very different. With stage hypnosis, the goal is to entertain an audience, and the needs and wishes of the volunteers who are hypnotized are usually ignored. Hypnotic subjects in stage hypnosis are often encouraged to act in ways that seem embarrassing, and they might feel used and ignored after the experience. The stage hypnotist does not seek to help subjects learn skills so they can feel more comfortable and in control in their daily lives. Stage hypnosis is all about entertainment at the expense of the hypnotic subjects.

On the other hand, with clinical hypnosis, the goal is to help you learn to use your natural hypnotic abilities to feel better. Clinical hypnosis aims to help you to reduce the intensity of pain, increase the ability to ignore pain, to have pain be less bothersome, to sleep better, and to get back to doing the activities that are most important to you. Hypnosis has been shown to help with each of these outcomes. Clinical hypnosis is all about helping you achieve what you wish.

People's response to all treatments, including hypnosis, is variable. Some people see substantial benefits right away; others might take longer to show improvement. Research shows, however, that it is the rare individual who reports no benefits from hypnosis and from learning self-hypnosis skills. In fact, as described in the previous chapter, the majority of patients report that they can learn to use hypnosis to experience periods of pain relief, and many report marked decreases in their daily pain that lasts for as long as the outcomes are measured. Almost all patients who learn self-hypnosis report that they get other benefits from hypnosis as well.

Hypnosis and Self-Hypnosis: What You Can Expect

In Chapter 3, *hypnosis* was defined as a procedure in which one person (the subject) is guided by another person (the hypnotist) to respond to suggestions for changes in sensations, thoughts, or behavior. *Self-hypnosis* was described as occurring when the subject enters the hypnotic trance state on his or her own, and then uses that state to feel better or to make behavior change easier.

Some people, especially those with a lot of hypnotic ability, have learned to use self-hypnosis on their own without any professional help. They have learned that they can become so absorbed in a hobby that they lose track of time—and can feel so relaxed and absorbed during this time that they do not notice anxiety, distress, or pain. Of course, this is one reason that people engage in hobbies. Hobbies can make people feel better, and allow them to experience some of the benefits of self-hypnosis.

Some people with very high levels of hypnotic skill report that there are times when they do not feel pain, even during medical procedures. For example, they may report that they do not require an anesthetic when they visit the dentist—they are able to just "go to the garden" or "zone out" during dental procedures. You do not need to have this very high level of hypnotic skill to benefit from hypnosis for pain management. But if you are one of the people who are already highly talented in this area, you will likely find hypnosis treatment to feel very "natural" to you.

Hypnosis Sessions

Most people learn self-hypnosis best by first experiencing hypnosis with an experienced clinician. With help and coaching, they can then learn to experience hypnosis on their own, and use this ability to maintain and build on the benefits they get from hypnotic treatment. At its most basic, a typical hypnosis session has three parts: (1) a hypnotic induction, (2) hypnotic suggestions, and (3) reorientation.

Hypnotic Induction

The induction is designed to help you enter a hypnotic state and increase your ability to respond to hypnotic suggestions. Just before the induction, the clinician may ask you to engage in a specific behavior (for example, to take a deep breath, hold it, and then let it go; or to touch your thumb to your middle finger). With each session, your mind learns more and more to associate the pre-induction behavior with entering a hypnotic state. It acts as a *cue* that you can use outside of the hypnosis session to induce self-hypnosis (more on this later).

Following the behavioral cue, the clinician will offer an induction. The induction almost always involves an invitation for you to focus your awareness and attention on a single experience. For example, the clinician may ask you to pay very close attention to a spot on a wall, or to listen very closely to his or her voice. The clinician might invite you to close your eyes and focus on your breathing, or suggest that you imagine being in a safe and comfortable place, and pay attention to what you see and experience in this place. These invitations to focus awareness can also be combined. For example, you may be invited to first pay attention to a spot on a wall, allow your eyes to close, focus on your breathing, and then "go" to a relaxing and safe place. The most important thing is that the objects or experiences you are invited to focus on are absorbing for you.

As you focus your attention on a single object or experience, changes happen in the activity in your brain. There is an increase in "slow" wave activity. If each neuron in your brain was like a single person in a world with billions of people, then as the people in this world focus their attention on an absorbing experience, many would stop talking. And those that continue to talk might do so much more quietly, and at a much slower rate. If you respond to the hypnotic induction, fewer neurons in your brain will fire and many of those that do will fire at a slower rate. The brain becomes more quiet and calm. This pattern of brain activity that is induced is much like that which occurs when people meditate by concentrating on a single object—say a candle or a mantra. Many people report that they feel both mentally relaxed and highly mentally clear in this state.

The other thing that happens as you relax and focus your attention is that the mind becomes more able to change how you feel—it become more flexible. To deepen your experience, the clinician may suggest additional experiences that you might create for yourself: sensations of heaviness or warmth in your limbs, or feeling even more relaxed and comfortable. Depending on your own hypnotic ability, you may feel deeply absorbed within just a minute or two, or you might need more time to feel pleasantly relaxed. Often as people become more experienced with hypnosis, it takes them less and less time to feel like they are in a hypnotic state.

Hypnotic Suggestions

Following the hypnotic induction, the clinician will offer suggestions for your brain to consider responding to. The clinician may add that your brain will respond only "to suggestions that are *appropriate for your comfort and well-being*," reminding your mind that it has control over which suggestions to respond to and which ones to ignore. The hypnotic suggestions offered will include any one or more of a very large number of possible suggestions for changes in your sensations, feelings, mood, thoughts, or behavior. The suggestions that are offered depend entirely on your treatment goals, goals that you and your clinician have agreed to work towards.

If you are using hypnosis for pain management, the suggestions will likely include a decrease in pain or its impact (for example, feeling less pain by imagining bathing the body part that is in pain in a healing and comforting liquid, closing the gate on pain input into the spine, not being bothered by pain, being able to ignore pain). But the suggestions may also include being able to distance yourself from the pain, changes in your thoughts about pain, or how you might choose to cope with pain. They may also include being able to be more active while also being more comfortable, or being able to get to sleep and stay asleep more easily.

After the primary suggestions are given, the clinician will usually offer what are called post-hypnotic suggestions: suggestions that the benefits you experienced during the hypnosis session will last beyond the session and (for as long as this is helpful and benefits you) become a permanent part of how your brain works. These suggestions are made so that you can experience the comfort of the hypnosis session as you go about the rest of your day. Because your brain is more open to responding to (appropriate) suggestions at this point, the clinician may also suggest that you will be able to enter this comfortable hypnotic state whenever you wish by using the behavioral cue established at the start of the session (e.g., take a deep breath, hold it, let it go).

Reorientation

After the last post-hypnotic suggestion, the clinician will likely invite you to reorient yourself, perhaps by suggesting that you will become "more awake and alert" with each number that is counted in a series. Or the clinician may suggest that you can allow yourself to become awake and alert at your own pace, perhaps cuing yourself that you are ready to end the session by allowing your eyes to open.

The hypnotic session can be just a few minutes long or may last for 30 minutes, an hour, or even longer. Brief sessions are excellent for giving you an opportunity to experience using hypnosis in a very short period of time. You may be like many other people and find substantial benefit from being able to engage in several very brief (1 to 3 minutes) self-hypnosis sessions during each day. Brief hypnosis sessions with a clinician can help you learn to do this.

Longer sessions can give you more time to enter a hypnotic state and make it possible to hear a number of different suggestions or hear the same suggestion many times, all of which can enhance the beneficial effects of the suggestions. How long the hypnosis session lasts will depend on the goals that you and your clinician have for the hypnosis component of the session.

Following the hypnotic session, the clinician will often invite you to share what you experienced. This is your opportunity to tell the clinician what you found to be most helpful and effective. Did you have enough time to enter a comfortably relaxed hypnotic state? Which parts of the induction did you like the most? Which parts could you do without? The more your clinician knows about your response, the more he or she will be able to make the next session even more helpful.

How Many Hypnosis Sessions Should You Have?

The research studies that have demonstrated hypnosis to be effective for chronic pain usually provide 4 to 10 hypnosis sessions. The exact number that is needed, however, has not yet been determined. It is reasonable to start with four treatment sessions, as that may be enough for you to improve your situation, obtain audio recordings for home use, and learn the self-hypnosis skills you can use to maintain your progress. On the other hand, you may determine that you are just getting started after four sessions, and could benefit from some additional sessions to address other treatment goals, or to build on benefits that are starting to emerge. In this case, you may elect to continue treatment with more sessions.

The overall goal of self-hypnosis is to allow you to recreate the beneficial effects that occur during your clinician-guided hypnosis sessions. These benefits include a global relaxed state that results in a type of brain activity associated with decreased pain. If pain relief is a goal, then spending 2 to 3 minutes each hour practicing self-hypnosis will not only increase your self-hypnosis skills, but may also allow you to experience less pain intensity and pain-related distress throughout the day.

The components and structure of your self-hypnosis sessions are basically the same as clinician-guided hypnosis sessions. Self-hypnosis thus includes an induction, suggestions, and reorientation. As you are learning self-hypnosis, it is best to do so in a place and time when there are very few distractions. It is also ideal if you practice self-hypnosis somewhere that you can be physically comfortable—a favorite chair, for example.

Because the brain state associated with hypnosis is similar to the state of the brain right *before* you go to sleep, you may find that on occasion you will fall asleep when you practice self-hypnosis. This tendency can be taken advantage of if you want to use your skills to help you get to sleep at night (see Chapter 9). However, your goals for using self-hypnosis during the day also likely include enhancing positive changes in your sensations, feelings, thoughts, and behavior. These changes can be difficult to establish if you are sleeping during your self-hypnosis sessions. Therefore, if you are finding that you are often going to sleep when you practice self-hypnosis, you may want to practice during times of the day when you might be less likely to fall asleep (for example, mid- to late morning, *before* lunch).

Also, you should avoid practicing self-hypnosis when it would be unsafe to do so—for example, while driving or operating machinery. Safe driving or use of machinery requires your undivided attention. Hypnosis, by encouraging you to focus your awareness and then respond to suggestions for change, is very absorbing.

Self-Hypnosis Induction

If you have an established behavioral cue that you engage in just before you start your hypnosis sessions with the clinician, you can begin your self-hypnosis induction with that cue. Getting comfortable in your chair, you can take a deep breath, hold it, perhaps for 10 seconds or so, and then let it go. Then notice how the focused state of awareness that you enter when you are having a hypnosis session with the clinician just seems to occur. At this point, you can use any one of the inductions presented in this workbook (see Chapter 6), or a self-hypnosis induction that your clinician has taught you.

Self-Hypnosis Suggestions

Following the induction, you will then read or make suggestions to yourself that you will experience changes in your pain (Chapter 7), thoughts (Chapter 8), or behavior and sleep (Chapter 9). The suggestions that you read or say to yourself can be planned by you or include ideas suggested by your clinician. Some individuals, especially those who practice self-hypnosis a great deal, find that they can enter the hypnotic state and then allow their mind to "find" or to "tell them" the suggestion that would be most appropriate at the time. Either way, you should take the time you want or need to be aware of, and then respond to, the suggestion or suggestions. Following this, you should allow yourself to shift to the reorientation and final phase of self-hypnosis.

Reorientation

Once you have completed the suggestion portion of the self-hypnosis session, you can allow yourself to reorient. This step allows you to bring your attention back to your day-to-day life. Two reorientation procedures you could use are presented in the final chapter of this workbook (Chapter 10), which gives some examples of complete self-hypnosis sessions. You may also develop a reorientation procedure yourself, or use one taught to you by your clinician.

How Often Should You Practice Self-Hypnosis?

Preliminary evidence from research suggests that patients who practice self-hypnosis more often report more benefits than those who practice less. This makes sense, if you consider self-hypnosis to be a skill like any other skill, such as golfing, playing the piano, or cooking. Researchers have not yet determined, however, if there is an "ideal" amount of practice. Certainly, it is possible to do too much—if you listen to an audio recording of your hypnosis sessions so frequently that you have no time to live your life. Alternatively, just listening to a recording or practicing self-hypnosis once a month would likely not be enough to produce benefit. In our research studies, we recommend that patients listen to the audio recordings once each day, and practice brief self-hypnosis two to six times every day. Following these recommendations will make it more likely that you will achieve the benefits that you wish. Ultimately, of course, it is you alone who will decide how often you want to practice, and you that will reap the rewards.

What You Should Tell the Clinician Working with You Prior to Choosing to Use Hypnosis

Prior to hypnosis treatment, you will meet with the clinician for a thorough evaluation of your pain problem. Together you will develop a treatment plan with specific treatment goals, and then discuss what treatment approaches you and your clinician think would work best to achieve your goals. These treatment goals may include reductions in how much pain you feel and how much pain bothers you. They will also likely include an increase in your ability to ignore pain, so that you can more easily focus on what is most important and meaningful to you. Other achievable goals might include an improvement in your day-to-day mood, activity level, and sleep quality. Hypnosis can help with all of these treatment goals, but hypnosis is not the only treatment that can do so. Your clinician may, in fact, recommend that treatment begin with non-hypnotic approaches that have been demonstrated to be effective, such as cognitive behavior therapy (CBT).

You can make the evaluation most useful by coming prepared. First, if you are taking any medications, you should write down the names and doses (and how often you take them) on a sheet of paper. You should also either have in mind, or write down if necessary, previous medications and treatments you have tried for pain. Third, you should bring your responses to the Helpful and Unhelpful Thoughts and Coping Questionnaires from Chapter 2. Be prepared to tell the clinician about any positive and negative significant events that have happened (or are happening) in your life.

Finally, it is important that you tell the clinician how you want your life to be different following treatment. For some patients, the only treatment goal they can envision is a reduction in pain. This is a reasonable goal, and achievable for many patients who receive hypnosis treatment and learn self-hypnosis—but it is rarely the only goal worth considering. To help you get the most out of the initial evaluation, and ultimately out of treatment, you should come prepared to discuss what other changes you want to make in your life. Even if treatment does not eliminate all of your pain, you can learn skills to help you minimize the impact of pain on your life, and get back to a life that brings you satisfaction and hope.

Chapter Summary

Many people do not have direct experience with hypnosis. What they believe may have been learned from what they have seen in the movies or television or on stage. Unfortunately, most of the information about clinical hypnosis from these sources is wrong. Hypnosis is not the same as sleep. It does not give another person "control" over the hypnotic subject. Moreover, response to hypnosis is unrelated to being "weak-minded" or gullible; virtually everyone is capable of responding to hypnosis and hypnotic suggestions. People do not usually lose conscious awareness during hypnosis, and you do not need to experience a "deep" level of focused attention to benefit from hypnosis. At the same time, you need not remember *everything* that occurred during a hypnosis session to benefit. Finally, clinical hypnosis is not like stage hypnosis. With clinical hypnosis, the goal and focus is to help the patient learn to use his or her imagination and attention to feel better. Clinical hypnosis seeks to give you skills that you will find useful for getting more control over your experience of pain and your emotional response to pain. The "side effects" of hypnosis, such as improved sleep and having more energy and an increased sense of well-being, can improve the overall quality of your life.

A typical hypnosis session includes three components: a hypnotic induction, hypnotic suggestions, and reorientation. When hypnosis is used for chronic pain management, the suggestions usually include post-hypnotic suggestions that the benefits achieved during the hypnosis session will last beyond the session. The goal with hypnosis is to help you make changes in the way your brain processes pain and pain-related thoughts, so you can feel better all of the time. To facilitate this, you can listen to audio recordings of the hypnosis sessions between your treatment sessions and long after treatment is over. In addition, your clinician may recommend that you practice self-hypnosis on your own, without the audio recordings. When you do, the components are the same as those for hypnosis: an induction followed by suggestions and then reorientation. You can practice and obtain the benefits of self-hypnosis for just 2 or 3 minutes at a time, several times during the day, or practice for longer, depending on your goals.

Most patients get the most out of hypnosis if they first learn it with the help of an experienced clinician. An important first step when working with a clinician is the initial evaluation. You should prepare for the initial evaluation by writing down all of the medications you are taking, and also bring your responses to the Helpful and Unhelpful Thoughts and Coping Questionnaires. It is also useful to come to the evaluation with an initial sense of what you want your treatment goals to be—how you want your life to be different. Towards the end of the initial evaluation you and your clinician should have developed a list of very specific treatment goals that you will work towards together. Based on these goals, the clinician will recommend which treatments to use. Although it is likely that hypnosis will be among them, it is not the only treatment option available.

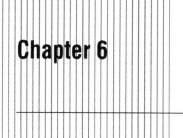

Chapter 6

Practicing Self-Hypnosis: Entering the Hypnotic "State"

Goals

■ To understand the purpose of a hypnotic induction

■ To learn and practice three hypnotic inductions that can be used for self-hypnosis

■ To learn how to "fine-tune" your hypnotic inductions to make them most effective

Chapter Overview

As mentioned in the previous chapter, hypnosis sessions almost always begin with an induction. This chapter describes the purpose of the induction, and then provides three basic inductions that you can use during self-hypnosis. It ends with a discussion about how you can keep track of your own responses to different inductions in order to get the most out of hypnosis and self-hypnosis.

What Is a Hypnotic Induction?

The hypnotic induction is the first step in any hypnosis procedure. It is based on a single very simple idea: when people focus their attention and become very absorbed on a single object, they become more able to change how they feel. The classic object of focus that has been used in many movies is a swinging pocket watch, but virtually any object or stimulus can be used. It can be a visual object like the pocket watch, a candle, or a spot on a wall. It can be something you hear, like the clinician's voice. Or it could be something that you feel, like your breathing. It could also be some image that you generate yourself, such as a beach scene or an image of some other safe and relaxing place.

When people focus their awareness in this way, changes happen in the brain. There is an overall decrease in activity—the brain calms down. During this experience, the part of the brain that keeps track of time can become so inactive that you might lose track of time. The nerve cells in the part of the brain that prompt feelings of worry or anxiety are less active, so you feel less anxious during and after a hypnotic induction. As a result of these brain activity changes, people often respond to hypnotic inductions by feeling more calm and relaxed, and yet more focused at the same time.

You may sometimes choose to use the induction to simply get into a hypnotic "state," given that you will likely find the state very comfortable. Entering this state has many positive health benefits on its own. Often, though, you will follow your self-guided induction with self-suggestions for changes in your experience of pain (Chapter 7), changes in your thoughts and mood (Chapter 8), or changes in your activity or sleep quality (Chapter 9).

Using the Inductions in this Chapter

This chapter describes three simple inductions that you can use to enter a hypnotic state. They are modeled on the inductions used in our research on hypnosis and chronic pain management—studies that support the efficacy of hypnosis treatment for chronic pain. Therefore, they can be viewed as inductions that have scientific support. That said, however, you and your clinician will likely find that you respond more strongly to some inductions than to others, and you may choose to modify these inductions to make them even more effective for you.

For each induction, the instructions are simple. First, read through the entire induction until you understand the steps. Then make a copy of the induction and hold it in your hand or place it on a clipboard in front of you while you are sitting in a very comfortable chair. Then simply slowly read each induction, and allow yourself to follow each step.

If you are practicing the induction on your own as a way to feel more relaxed and comfortable, you can simply read the induction and enjoy the experience of the state you create for yourself for as long as you would like. In this case, you can allow yourself to "return" from the hypnotic state when you are ready. If you are going to follow the induction with self-suggestions for changes in pain, mood, sleep quality, or behavior, then you can enjoy the hypnotic state you create for yourself, and *then* move on to reading a script from the chapters that follow for the self-suggestions you wish to make.

Basic Countdown Induction

The instructions for the basic countdown induction are presented on pages 78–79. Notice that this induction, like all of the others in this workbook, begins with a specific cue: to take a deep and satisfying breath, hold it for a moment (usually about 5–10 seconds), and then let it go. It is a good idea to begin each induction with a cue such as this. If you do this, you will associate the cue with your own hypnotic response.

In the countdown induction presented on pages 78–79, the deep breath cue is used at each step. It takes advantage of the fact that there is a natural relaxation response that follows an exhalation. Thus, each breath can contribute more to your feelings of relaxation, helping to create a deep sense of overall relaxation by the end of the induction. When using the breathing cue, it is best to hold your breath for long enough so that you feel ready to let it go, but not so long that you ever feel uncomfortable. Let yourself find the timing that works best for you.

Once you have practiced this induction several times while reading the instructions on pages 78–79, you might have memorized enough of it to practice it on your own without the instructions.

When you do so, you can allow your eyes to close at any point, and then imagine yourself going down an elevator into "deeper" levels of comfort with every number you count, or imagine the numbers appearing in your mind's eye each time you count a number to yourself. Using your ability to picture yourself in an elevator or picture the numbers appearing in front of you will enhance the effects of the induction.

Once you reach the number 10, you can then enjoy the feelings of relaxation that you have created for yourself for as long as you wish. Just a couple of minutes would be fine if you are taking a short break. Many patients choose to stay in this state for 5 or 10 minutes, as they find it so calming and relaxing. As mentioned above, you can also use this, or any of the other three inductions presented in this chapter, as a precursor to one or more self-suggestions in the chapters that follow.

Also, you need not worry about getting "stuck" in a hypnotic state. You should find that the state of focused awareness that you can achieve with this and other inductions feels very familiar to you. It is much like the state you get into whenever you feel very relaxed and focused, such as sitting on a beach watching a sunset while on vacation, or engaging in some interesting and absorbing hobby. You might sometimes lose track of time in these situations, but you do not get "stuck" in them. When it is time for you to return to your usual day-to-day state of mind, you will do so.

Relaxation Induction

Another induction commonly used in hypnosis treatment for pain management focuses on suggestions for relaxation (see pages 80–81). One of the reasons that these inductions are so useful is that many people are able to respond to relaxation suggestions. Almost everyone experiences moments of physical relaxation at some point in their lives; for example, most people feel relaxed just before going to sleep at night. Another reason that relaxation inductions and relaxation suggestions are so useful for individuals with chronic pain is that the feeling of relaxation, and the mental calm that often accompanies this feeling, is inconsistent with the suffering sometimes associated with pain. Patients with chronic pain who are able to learn to experience relaxation whenever they wish are often able to feel less pain, and less distress associated with their pain.

When practicing the induction on pages 80–81, it is best to read the script slowly and give yourself time to follow each suggestion as you read it. The whole exercise should take 10 minutes or longer. If you finish reading the induction in less than this amount of time, you are probably reading it too quickly, and not taking the time needed to experience each suggestion. You should ideally plan to allow at least 10 seconds—more if possible—to elapse between each sentence. As you read the induction suggestions, really give yourself the time to *experience* the feelings of relaxation that you allow yourself to imagine.

As with the countdown induction, once you have practiced the relaxation induction a number of times, you can move on to practicing it without reading the script. When doing this, simply allow your mind to move from one body part to the next, letting each body part feel relaxed before moving on. Notice the specific sensations that *you* feel as your body relaxes. Is it heaviness, warmth, lightness, a slight tingling, something else? Whatever the sensations are for you, you should pay attention to those sensations and allow them to grow.

"Safe Place" Induction

The final induction is the "safe place" induction (see pages 82–83). This induction takes advantage of many people's ability to imagine themselves in a specific location, and picture in their mind's eye the details of that place. If you can imagine yourself in a place where you feel very safe and comfortable, then feelings of relaxation and comfort will naturally follow the images that you create.

Safe place inductions and suggestions are particularly useful for individuals who have a talent for imagery, and who are able to visualize a place in enough detail so that the feelings associated with the place are elicited automatically. It is also useful to include all of the senses when imagining the safe place. To smell the smells (for example, the salty air if it is at a beach), hear the sounds (for example, the rush of water if it is in a meadow next to a mountain stream), and feel the textures (for example, of sand or dirt if it is outside) and temperature. You may find that some senses help you to experience yourself as being in your safe place more easily than other sensations. If so, it would be wise to focus on those senses as you enter your place and experience yourself being there.

As you gain more experience in using the safe place induction, you will find it easier to allow yourself to be pleasantly surprised at what you can see, hear, smell, and touch. To make the exercise most effective, it is best to allow your mind to create the scene for you rather than to "work" at creating it for yourself.

If you are using the safe place induction to simply experience the benefits of a hypnotic induction, and you do not plan to move on to giving yourself suggestions for changes in pain, mood, activity, or sleep quality, you could stay in the safe place for as long as you wish. Just 2 or 3 minutes might be long enough to produce a general calming of brain activity. The benefits of these changes—feeling more relaxed and calm—will likely spill over into the minutes and hours after the practice session.

Your Unique Response to Hypnotic Inductions

Your response to different hypnotic inductions will be unique. For these reasons, and to make sure that you get the most out of each possible induction, it is important to tailor the inductions to fit your responses. Tailoring inductions is easy: all you need to do is notice how well you respond to the inductions that you use, and focus on the components of the induction that you respond well to. If there is a part of the induction that you do not like for any reason at all, you can simply ignore that part. You should also discuss your responses to these inductions, and any others that your clinician suggests you try, directly with your clinician. Together, you will be able to modify the inductions to best fit how you respond.

When evaluating an induction, notice (1) how long it takes you to get into a very relaxed and focused hypnotic state, (2) the specific types of induction (e.g., countdown, relaxation, safe place) that you respond to the best, and (3) the type of senses that are easiest for you to manipulate and experience (smell, sight, hearing, touch, taste, temperature).

Your clinician will probably provide you with inductions that take anywhere from just a few minutes to up to 10 or more minutes. As you experience these inductions you will very likely have a strong sense of the length of induction that works best for you. Following each session, you should tell the clinician if you would like the next induction to be longer, shorter, or about the same time.

Individuals also differ with respect to the *type* of inductions they respond to best. Although many individuals find relaxation inductions to be among the easiest, there are also individuals who say that they are "unable to relax" and who therefore struggle with inductions that invite them to feel relaxed. These individuals may find the safe place induction to be much more effective. If neither of these produces satisfactory results, then your clinician can work with you to find an induction or two that you do respond to. It is important to remember, though, that you need not enter a "deep" state of hypnosis to respond to suggestions for changes in pain or other pain-related variables. A light state of relaxed focus is usually quite adequate. The key is to find the suggestions that will result in you feeling this state of comfortable focus.

Finally, individuals seem to differ with respect to the senses that they can most easily imagine and create for themselves. Some people are able to create visual images easily and naturally. These are the individuals who would likely respond well to the safe place induction, which takes advantage of people's ability to visualize environments. Other people are able to imagine specific physical sensations. They can easily imagine their hand in a tub of warm water or imagine a sense of muscles feeling relaxed, of limbs feeling heavy or light. If you are one of these people, then the inductions you are given and practice should include frequent references to physical sensations.

To help you to understand how you are responding to the different inductions that you try, and to help you communicate this understanding to your clinician, you should complete the Induction Response Form on pages 84–85 for each induction that you try. The form has space for you to communicate your responses regarding the length of the induction, your overall response to the induction, and the specific components of the induction that you found most (and least) helpful. Your completed Induction Response Form can be used to inform your clinician, and together you can use this information to create an induction that will be just right for you.

Chapter Summary

A hypnotic induction is provided at the beginning of a hypnosis session to facilitate a relaxed and focused state of awareness. This state of awareness is a natural response to being absorbed in a stimulus or activity. Almost everyone experiences this state at some time in his or her daily life, so the state may seem very familiar to you. The state an individual experiences during and following an induction also appears to be essentially the same as the state associated with meditation, and this can be beneficial in and of itself. For this reason, you may choose to practice self-inductions just to feel relaxed.

Virtually any absorbing activity can induce the state of focused awareness associated with hypnosis. Three such activities were introduced in this chapter. They mirror the inductions that have been used in recent clinical trials of hypnosis for chronic pain management, and so represent inductions that have scientific support for their efficacy. However, there are many more inductions used by clinicians working in this area. You should pay attention to your response to the inductions that you and your clinician try (using the Induction Response Form), and discuss those responses with your clinician.

Together, you will be able to develop one or several inductions that take just the right amount of time and that help you to achieve a relaxed and focused state. When in this state, you will be in a better position to make changes you want to make in how you feel, behave, and think.

Countdown Induction Script

Just settle back and allow yourself to sit as comfortably as you can right now. Go ahead and adjust yourself to the most comfortable position. Take whatever time you need.

And notice how it is possible to increase your comfort, right now. Take a deep, satisfying breath and hold it just for a moment . . . Now let it go. And let yourself notice how good that feels.

In a moment, you will to count from 1 to 10. As you count each number, take a deep, satisfying breath, hold it . . . and then let it all the way out. And as you count each number, you can imagine that you feel yourself settling down, one level of comfort at a time, into a deeper and deeper experience of comfort and relaxation. Perhaps you will imagine yourself going down an elevator; perhaps you will picture each number as you count. Either is fine. With each number you count, just allow yourself to settle down into a deeper and deeper experience of comfort and relaxation. So that, when you reach the tenth level, you can really enjoy an experience of deep, comfortable ease.

One. One level down into deeper comfort. And now take another deep, satisfying breath. Hold it . . . and then let it all the way out.

Two. Two levels down. That's right. And then, another deep, satisfying breath.

Three. Three levels down. And now you may already notice yourself feeling more comfortable. Notice different parts of the body that are relaxing or feeling heavier. Picturing each number as you count. And then take another deep breath.

Four. Four levels down. Maybe noticing a deep, relaxing, and restful heaviness in your forehead. Feeling it beginning to spread. Across the eyes, across the face, into the jaw. Deep, restful, heavy. When ready, take another deep breath. Hold it, and let it go.

Five. Halfway down, and already beginning, perhaps, to really enjoy this opportunity to feel relaxed, comfortable, and at ease. And when you are ready to feel even more comfortable, take another deep breath. Hold it for a moment, and let it go. Really notice the relaxation.

Six. Six levels down. Perhaps noticing that the sounds around you are sounds that can become more and more a part of your experience of comfort and well-being, with nothing to bother you or disturb you as we continue. And take another deep breath, hold it . . . and let it go.

Seven. Seven levels down. Right now, there is nothing you have to do. Nothing required of you and no one you have to please. No one else you have to take care of. Just this opportunity to feel deeply comfortable and at ease. Really let this sink in, and then when you are ready, take another deep and satisfying breath. Hold it. And let it go.

Eight. Eight levels down. Allowing this opportunity to become more and more absorbed by your experience of comfort and well-being. Another deep breath.

Nine. Nine levels down . . . Perhaps noticing that, as your body relaxes more and more deeply, your whole body feels as if it were becoming heavier and heavier. Really sinking deeper and deeper into the comfort of the chair. And one more deep breath.

And then ten. The tenth level of relaxation. Notice, now, how deeply comfortable, how very much at ease you can feel.

Just settle back and allow yourself to sit as comfortably as you can right now. Go ahead and adjust yourself to the most comfortable position. Take whatever time you need.

And notice how it is possible to increase your comfort, right now. Take a deep, satisfying breath and hold it just for a moment . . . Now let it go. And let yourself notice how good that feels.

And now, allow your whole body to relax. Allow all your muscles to go limp. Give yourself the time you need to let this happen.

And then allow special muscle groups to relax even more. Starting with your right hand. Imagine that all the muscles and tendons in the right hand are relaxing. As the hand relaxes, be aware of any sensations that let you know that the hand feels more relaxed. Perhaps a sense of warmth, or of heaviness; whatever sensation that lets you know that your right hand is becoming more and more relaxed, limp, heavy, warm, and comfortable.

And allow that relaxation to spread. Up into the wrist. The forearm, elbow, and upper arm. The whole arm becoming more relaxed and heavy. Any tension draining away, as the arm feels heavier, and heavier, almost as if it were made of lead. So comfortable, so relaxed.

Now allow your awareness to move to your left hand. Imagine how the left hand is becoming limp, heavy, and relaxed, heavier and heavier. Any tension just draining away. Let yourself be aware of any sensation that lets you know that the left hand is relaxing. A warmth, a heaviness. And allow the relaxation to spread. Up the wrist and into the arm. The whole left arm relaxing, heavier and heavier.

As you continue to allow both arms to feel more and more relaxed, you can be aware that the relaxation continues to spread. Into the shoulders. All the muscles in the shoulders letting go, relaxing, letting all the tension drain out of the shoulders. Feeling so relaxed, heavy, comfortable.

And the relaxation continues to spread. Into the neck. All the muscles and tendons of the neck letting go, one by one. Just allowing the head to rest, as you feel more and more comfortable, more and more at ease. The whole body becoming relaxed, very relaxed, calm and peaceful. Allowing the feelings of comfortable relaxation to spread up around the ears, letting all the tension drain away, the muscles around the eyes letting go, relaxing, as do the muscles in the face and jaw. Limp, relaxed, comfortable, and at peace.

It feels so good to take a vacation from stress, as the relaxation continues, down the back, into the chest, the stomach, and pelvis. As the body relaxes, so too does the mind relax. Feeling calm and confident.

And the relaxation continues to spread. Down into the legs. The right leg, feeling so very heavy, comfortable. Any tension draining out. Limp, heavy, and comfortable. And then the left leg, any tension draining out of the left leg, to be replaced by comfort. A heavy, pleasant comfortable and deep relaxation.

The whole body relaxing. And when it feels as if you are as relaxed as you can be, take a moment to allow yourself to relax *even more,* becoming even *more* relaxed. More comfortable, without a care in the world.

Just settle back and allow yourself to sit as comfortably as you can right now. Go ahead and adjust yourself to the most comfortable position. Take whatever time you need.

And notice how it is possible to increase your comfort, right now. Take a deep, satisfying breath and hold it just for a moment . . . Now let it go. And let yourself notice how good that feels.

And now allowing yourself to drift off, you can imagine yourself in a wonderful, beautiful, and very safe place. As you step into your safe place, comfortable place, you notice a sense of relief. A sense of deep physical and emotional comfort. It is like a vacation from stress. You can really let go, knowing that you are so very safe. With nothing to bother you, and nothing to disturb you. Take your time to really *be* in this place now. Take as long as you need.

This is your time . . . a time to charge your batteries . . . You step into the place and can feel the ground or floor against your feet. If it is a beach, as you step onto the sand, and can feel its warmth on your feet . . . actually feel that warm sand . . . the texture . . . If it is a meadow, you can feel the firm ground below.

And as you look around . . . everything is so beautiful. Looking into the sky, you can see that it is incredibly blue . . . as blue a sky as you have ever seen . . . and if there are clouds, they are just floating there . . . so easily . . . white and fluffy . . . they look as relaxed as you feel . . .

There is nothing, nothing at all that you *have* to do here. No one you have to please, no one to take care of.

And you can smell the air . . . and hear the sounds that are associated with your place. The sounds that you associate with feeling so relaxed and so free.

Perhaps there are plants. And you can focus on the leaves. They are so green, perhaps waving a little in the breeze, feeling the breeze against your skin. The temperature is just right . . . just right for feeling so relaxed, and yet so focused.

And in front of you, you can see a soaking tub of water. It is as if it were built just for you. You know that it fits you just right . . . and you know that the healing water in this tub can make you feel even better . . . even more relaxed, comfortable, and strong.

You might decide to allow yourself to move to the tub, to sit back, feeling the support of a built-in chair, supporting your head above the water. And the water just *feels* so good. It, too, is just the right *temperature*. The perfect amount of warmth or coolness. You can actually feel the water all around your body, breathing so naturally and easily with your head supported.

Maybe noticing how the healing liquid seems to *soak into* areas of the body that could benefit from feeling better, stronger, and more energized. Of course, you know that this state of focused awareness is so healthy for you. It strengthens your immune system, it relaxes you and gives you more energy, it allows the mind to relax and yet feel more focused at the same time.

You might enjoy just letting yourself go, and allow your mind and body to heal, as you experience a timeless feeling of relaxation.

Induction Response Form

Date: _____   Induction used: _____

The length of the induction was (check one):

    ( ) Too short

    ( ) About right

    ( ) Too long

Overall, my response to the induction was:

    ( ) Very positive; I felt very relaxed and focused following the induction

    ( ) Somewhat positive; I felt somewhat relaxed and focused following the induction

    ( ) Neutral; I did not feel particularly relaxed or focused following the induction

    ( ) Somewhat negative; I felt a little more tense and less focused following the induction

    ( ) Very negative; I was distracted and frustrated following the induction

The components of the induction that seemed most helpful were (list each one):

_____

_____

_____

The components of the induction that seemed less helpful were (list each one):

_____

_____

_____

The things I *saw* during the induction included: _____

The things I *felt* during the induction included: _____

The things I *smelled* during the induction included: _____

The things I *heard* during the induction included: _____

The things I *tasted* during the induction included: _____

Which senses were most vivid for you (select all that apply)?

( ) Sight

( ) Touch

( ) Internal feelings (feeling relaxed, warm, or heavy/light)

( ) Smell

( ) Hearing

( ) Taste

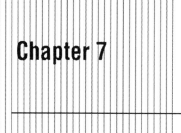

Chapter 7

Using Self-Hypnosis for Pain and Fatigue Management

Goal

- To learn and practice seven hypnotic suggestions for pain and fatigue management

Chapter Overview

This chapter presents seven suggestions that you can use to help your brain process information so that you experience less pain and fatigue. If you are working with a clinician who is using the treatment protocol outlined in the therapist guide that accompanies this patient workbook, the suggestions presented here will be familiar to you. You will have heard some or all of them in your treatment sessions, and should have audio recordings of the sessions to listen to at home. You can also use the scripts in this chapter on your own without audio recordings. Practice will enhance the efficacy of your treatment and give you even more control over your symptoms.

Practicing Self-Hypnosis

You already know that it is possible to influence your pain by changing activity in the different parts of the brain that process pain information. The six pain-focused suggestions presented in this chapter are designed to influence different areas of the nervous system that are involved in your experience of pain. A seventh suggestion targets fatigue, which accompanies pain for many individuals. Because you will likely respond more positively to some of the suggestions than others, it is recommended that you practice each one at least several times, and then determine which suggestions work best for you.

Those that result in your feeling better for longer can be memorized with repeated use, and you can then use self-hypnosis whenever you wish—even several times a day for just a few minutes at a time—to obtain the most benefit.

The suggestion scripts presented in this chapter are designed to (1) reduce pain intensity, (2) decrease how much pain bothers you, (3) replace painful sensations with more pleasant or neutral ones, (4) produce pain relief ("analgesia") in specific areas of the body, (5) help you to feel deeply relaxed, (6) reduce the frequency and severity of breakthrough pain, and (7) reduce the severity and impact of fatigue.

As a first step, make photocopies of all of the suggestions that you plan to try. Then pick the first one that interests you, and place it in a clipboard or hold it in your hand while sitting in your favorite comfortable chair. Next, induce self-hypnosis using one of the inductions presented in Chapter 6, or perhaps a separate induction you have developed with your clinician.

Following the self-hypnosis induction, you should be in a relaxed yet focused state of awareness. At this point, read (slowly) the chosen pain or fatigue management script. After doing so, give yourself time to notice the effects and benefits of the self-hypnosis session you just completed. Later in the day, complete the Response to Self-Hypnosis Questionnaire provided at the end of the chapter.

You may choose to try a different suggestion each day, or to use the same script several days in a row to enhance its effects before trying a new one. Either method will help you learn which scripts are most helpful for you and your pain problem. At your next session with your clinician, you should bring all of the Response to Self-Hypnosis Questionnaire forms you completed for discussion.

Pain Reduction

A hypnotic suggestion script that targets pain reduction is presented on pages 94–95. The suggestions contained in this script target multiple components of pain. When reading the suggestions to yourself, it is important to notice any changes in your sensations and images in response to the text. For example, when the script invites you to imagine any painful or uncomfortable sensations as an image, allow an image that represents the pain to appear in your mind's eye, whatever it may be. And then watch in your mind's eye as that image changes and drifts away.

The paragraphs at the end of the script are post-hypnotic suggestions to extend the benefits that you created during your self-hypnosis session beyond the session. The final paragraph contains reorienting suggestions that will help you to enjoy the feelings you have created, and to "come back" in your own time and when you are ready. Once you have reoriented, you can proceed with whatever else you have planned for the day. At some point following the self-hypnosis session, perhaps several hours later when you have had a chance to notice and think about your response, you should complete the Response to Self-Hypnosis Questionnaire. Bring this and other completed forms with you to your next treatment session.

Decreased Pain Unpleasantness

You already know that pain has different components, and that each of these components is processed in different parts of the brain. This explains why it is possible to sometimes feel a little pain and perhaps be very upset and bothered by it, while at other times is it possible feel a great deal of pain and somehow feel much less bothered. The possibility that one can feel some pain and still be happy and content makes it important to include suggestions to help make this happen.

The script presented on pages 96–97 was written to target the emotional or unpleasantness component of pain. It reminds you that it is possible to feel a kind of detachment or "acceptance" of painful sensations. Paradoxically, as you practice and allow yourself to "accept" pain as it is, you may notice that its intensity decreases. This occurs because the area of the brain that processes information about your emotional response to pain (the ACC) can influence the part of the brain that processes information about the intensity of pain (the sensory cortices; see Chapter 1). As your ACC becomes less active, so can activity in the sensory cortices, causing your experience of pain to decrease.

Sensory Substitution

Sensory substitution suggestions are designed to help your brain focus more on comfortable and neutral sensations, thereby decreasing the focus on and experience of pain. For protective reasons, and left on its own, the brain will tend to focus more on sensations that it determines are indications of threat to our health and well-being. That is the reason that pain sensations can be so distracting. Helping the brain to become more aware of less painful and distressing symptoms can effectively calm down the whole brain, leaving you with lower levels of daily pain. A script that you can use for sensory substitution can be found on pages 98–99.

Hypnotic Analgesia

Another common suggestion made during hypnotic treatment of chronic pain is "hypnotic analgesia." In response to this suggestion, you imagine a powerful analgesic soaking into the previously painful area (see script on pages 100–101). This suggestion is similar in many ways to the "anesthetic arm" suggestion used in the study described in Chapter 4. As you recall, the subjects in this study were given the hypnotic suggestion that one arm was "vulnerable" and the other was "anesthetic." When both arms were exposed to high levels of heat, the heat produced less inflammatory responses in the "anesthetic" arm, and there were fewer chemicals released in the skin of the "anesthetic" arm that make nerves sensitive to pain. Hypnotic analgesia suggestions, like those presented in the script on pages 100–101, may therefore be especially helpful for patients who have pain related to inflammatory responses (for example, arthritis pain) or who have pain in very focused areas (for example, the low back).

Deep Relaxation

Many people find it relatively easy to respond to suggestions for feeling relaxed. This is one reason that relaxation hypnotic inductions are used so often in hypnotic treatments of chronic pain. Also, for many people, the experience of feeling deeply relaxed is inconsistent with the experience of suffering; relaxation suggestions can therefore be used for pain management. See pages 102–103 for an example of a script suggesting deep relaxation.

One of the strengths of relaxation suggestions is their flexibility. Once you have memorized the script from multiple readings, you can develop your own very brief (1 or 2 minutes), moderately long (10 minutes), or very long (20 minutes or more) versions to use. The very brief version could be used many times throughout a day and could consist simply of engaging your hypnosis cue (deep breath, hold it, let it go) followed by an awareness of relaxation washing over you, moving up your arms, into your shoulders, and down the rest of the body. A moderately long version would consist of the script presented on pages 102–103, as written. If you respond well to this technique and want to experience an extremely deep sense of relaxation, you can take more time to notice how each body part is relaxing as you move through the body.

Because the deep relaxation script is essentially the same as the relaxation induction script, you may elect to use an induction that is not relaxation-focused when using the deep relaxation script on pages 102–103; for example, the countdown or safe place induction from Chapter 6. Alternatively, if you chose, you could use the relaxation induction from Chapter 6, and then simply deepen your experience of relaxation further by reading and responding to the suggestions presented in the deep relaxation script.

Reduced Breakthrough Pain

Breakthrough pain can be defined as pain that comes on suddenly, seemingly on its own without any cause, and that lasts for short periods of time. This type of pain can occur with many pain problems, although it tends to be most common in individuals with phantom limb pain (pain perceived as being in an arm or leg that has been amputated) or pain associated with cancer. The script presented on pages 104–105 provides suggestions that you may find helpful for managing this type of pain.

Fatigue Management

Feelings of fatigue are very common in individuals who have chronic pain. There are also some research reports suggesting that hypnosis can help individuals with fatigue feel more energy. The suggestions contained in the script presented on pages 106–107 are designed to help you "recharge" yourself and feel more energy when you wish.

Chapter Summary

The suggestions described in this chapter are designed to help you experience more comfort, more energy, and less pain. You will likely find that you respond better to some than to others, although it is not possible to predict with certainty which ones will work the best for you. It therefore makes sense to try each of the scripts at least once. You should note your responses using the Response to Self-Hypnosis form provided after the scripts following this chapter. Based on your responses, you will soon learn which suggestions are most helpful. As you practice reading the scripts, you will eventually memorize the critical components and be able to use them without having to read them.

In combination with the hypnotic suggestions you hear during your treatment sessions, and the repetition of those suggestions as you listen to audio recordings of the sessions, your self-hypnosis sessions should result in an increased ability to experience periods of pain relief and comfort. However, rarely if ever should you limit yourself to using *only* suggestions for pain or fatigue management. Hypnosis and self-hypnosis can also be used to improve your overall mood and well-being (Chapter 8) and make it easier for you to engage in activities that are most important to you and improve your sleep (Chapter 9).

Pain Reduction Script begins on the next page

With every breath you take, breathing comfort in and breathing discomfort out, you can wonder how you can be feeling . . . more and more comfortable, right here and now. You may be pleased, of course, but you may also be surprised that it's so much easier now to simply *focus on relaxation and comfort.* So easy to enjoy the relaxing, peaceful comfort of each breath. So simple, so natural, to attend to your breathing.

And at the same time, you can notice, almost as a side effect, that any uncomfortable feelings are drifting farther and farther away. You might even imagine these feelings as an image. Perhaps as leaves on a stream. Or as a fire burning on a piece of wood, or even as some other image floating on a log or piece of wood on the stream. You can actually see them. I don't know what the image is, but you do. You can see details, watching the image change. Perhaps floating, slowly drifting down the stream. Or if it is a fire, watching the fire burning out. Either way, the image is getting smaller and smaller. Disappearing.

And now, maybe you can take whatever image you have of the uncomfortable sensations, and imagine, in your mind's eye, lowering the image into a strongbox with a secure lid. Into the box the feelings go. And you can see yourself shutting the lid and securing it. Muffling the sensations. And then putting this box into a second very secure box, and shutting the lid. The sensations are in there, but muffled, quiet. And putting this second box into yet a third box. Shutting the lid. Securing it. Nothing can get out. And then, and you can use your creativity here, imagine sending the box far, far away. Maybe deep into space. Maybe across the ocean. But really picture it going away. Far, far away. So much easier to ignore now.

And with those sensations so far away, it is even easier to feel the comfort of every breath. So easy to let yourself daydream about a peaceful place, to imagine a happy time in your life or a happy time you'd like to have. Letting yourself feel free, right now, to just let your mind wander over pleasant memories and sensations.

Such a pleasure to be here, with nothing to bother you and nothing to disturb you. With every breath you take, breathing comfort in and tension or discomfort out, just notice how naturally you feel more and more comfort. And any feelings of discomfort seem to have lessened and maybe even disappeared altogether. Like some memory long forgotten. Or something you have stored away but is no longer a part of your awareness. Letting each breath you take contribute to your comfort and well-being.

You know, of course, that *any* sensations of comfort that you now feel are sensations that you have created for yourself. These sensations are within your power to create. And they can stay with you, if this would be helpful to you. They can last beyond the session, for minutes, hours, days, and even years. They can become a permanent part of what your mind gives to you at all times. As natural as breathing. Any benefits from your self-hypnosis are becoming an automatic part of who you are.

And now, if you wish, you can allow your eyes to close and enjoy the state you are in for as long as would like. Taking the time you need to come back to the here and now. When you are ready to come back to the here and now, you can signal to yourself that you are ready by allowing your eyes to open. And when they do, you will be comfortable and alert . . . ready to go on to do whatever it is that you would like to do next.

As you sink deeper into comfort, you can be aware of just how well you can feel, with nothing to bother you, and nothing to disturb you. It is possible for you to notice, right now, that even though the body provides input into the mind, it is the mind that creates sensations. And these sensations are always changing. They wax and wane, like all natural processes.

But this is not what is most important right now. What is important is this: that you are able to simply accept any sensations the mind creates just as they are. They come, they go. But you do not have to do anything about them. You can experience the sensations almost as if they were happening to someone else, or a different version of you. From a distance. Just notice them with an emotional detachment. Perhaps a curiosity about how they might change, but knowing that whatever sensations there are, *they do not have to bother you.*

Isn't it interesting how the sensations that we experience, and our emotional reaction to them, are different things? The sensations are one thing. Our emotional reaction is another. We can experience small sensations and have large emotions about them, or experience large sensations and be detached; hardly any emotion at all. It is possible to have a calm, warm, comfortable acceptance of our sensations; they simply are what they are. And notice how calming and reassuring this realization is. It can feel physically relaxing. A kind of letting go, not having to worry or bother anymore about these sensations, whatever they are. Freeing you up to think about the things in your life that are most important.

Many people are surprised to find that it becomes easier to relax the more they practice these skills. To feel relaxed and calm, no matter what is happening physically. I wonder if you will be surprised to find that you can experience this too. It might help to remember that you have the ability to take good care of your health as you need to. If there's any change in your feelings or sensations, your mind can notice this, and you will be able to take care of yourself as needed. But this can be done from a detached, calm, relaxing perspective. No matter what type of sensations you have, you really don't need to feel bothered by them.

Because with any of the old feelings, you know that you don't need to do anything at all about them. Just calmly accept them. It's just so satisfying and freeing to notice that, for some reason, all the sensations you can feel, all the feelings you notice, can become more and more a part of your experience of comfort and well-being, with nothing to bother you and nothing to disturb you. Although you can notice feelings and sensations, from a distance, there are no feelings that bother you or to disturb you right now.

You know that *any* feelings of detachment and acceptance that you experience are feelings that you have created for yourself; they are within your power to create. And they can stay with you. They can last beyond the session, for minutes, hours, days, and even years. They can become a permanent part of what your mind gives to you. As natural as breathing. The benefits from your self-hypnosis are becoming an automatic part of who you are.

And now, if you wish, you can allow your eyes to close and enjoy the state you are in for as long as would like. Taking the time you need to come back to the here and now. When you are ready to come back to the here and now, you can signal to yourself that you are ready by allowing your eyes to open. And when they do, you will be comfortable and alert . . . ready to go on to do whatever it is that you would like to do next.

You are aware that there are feelings and sensations that are very pleasant for you. It would be useful to imagine what they might be. Perhaps feelings of warmth are most pleasant, or a sense of strength, or a relaxing heaviness.

And you might wonder where in your body you are feeling the most comfort. Take a moment to really pay attention to that part of your body, and notice the feelings that the nerves there are sending to your brain. As you pay close attention to those feelings, you can notice that they are building and increasing, spreading. And as these sensations are noticed, as they build, you probably feel more and more calm, peaceful, and more and more relaxed.

You are training your nervous system so that it is possible to be more aware of pleasant sensations and helpful feelings, so much more aware of pleasant sensations and feelings, in fact, that it is hard to notice any other type of feelings. Noticing, just noticing, how your mind focuses more and more on these feelings of calmness, comfort, and relaxation.

In fact, your nerves are sending all kinds of interesting feelings to your brain all the time, and your brain can learn to filter out some sensations, and become increasingly absorbed in new, more comfortable feelings. As you pay attention to this, you can start to notice interesting feelings that are pleasant for you, in any areas of the body that you want to feel more comfortable.

And now you can relax further and allow these other feelings to grow, to expand, to take up more and more of your attention, so that your mind is less and less able to be aware of any other feelings. I wonder if you might be curious about just how absorbed you can become in noticing these comfortable and pleasant sensations and feelings. How good this feels. And your ability to do this is growing, and becoming more and more automatic all the time. Not only that, but the more you notice these good feelings, the better you feel emotionally . . . calmer and calmer . . . more and more hopeful and confident . . . You can just . . . feel *good*.

You know that any sense of noticing more comfortable feelings is an ability that you have. An ability that you are letting your mind practice. And any feelings that you are noticing can stay with you, and linger beyond the session. They can last for minutes, hours, days, and even years. The more you practice, the more they can become a permanent part of what your mind gives to you. As natural as breathing. The benefits from your self-hypnosis are becoming an automatic part of who you are.

And now, if you wish, you can allow your eyes to close and enjoy the state you are in for as long as would like. Taking the time you need to come back to the here and now. When you are ready to come back to the here and now, you can signal to yourself that you are ready by allowing your eyes to open. And when they do, you will be comfortable and alert . . . ready to go on to do whatever it is that you would like to do next.

As you know, an analgesic is a powerful medicine used to help you feel more comfortable. You are now going to use your imagination to anesthetize any areas that you would like to feel more comfortable.

You can imagine this analgesic any way you like: as a feeling of warmth, or coolness, or other sensation that is comfortable and perhaps a little interesting; or as a color, even as a powerful liquid medicine. However it feels right for you.

Now imagine the areas that you would like to feel more comfortable being completely surrounded and completely filled with a sensation of analgesia. A pleasant sensation of comfort. Picture these feelings spreading through that area. Notice how naturally, how easily, the analgesic can make those areas feel curiously different and much more pleasant, and even decreasing sensations from that area, as if it were disappearing.

Notice how easily you can feel those pleasant sensations just wash over everything. Notice how the analgesic sensations absorb and block out any discomfort. Such a pleasure to be able to imagine—to make real—such comfort. These areas of your body feeling more and more comfortable as the anesthesia spreads.

This powerful and long-lasting analgesic is doing its job. It has such positive effects. Greater comfort. A sense of calmness and of confidence. And it can last for hours. And, you might be very surprised, even days. As you gain more experience, this analgesic becomes more powerful and effective, and can last for as long as you need.

Your ability to use this analgesic is growing, and becoming a part of who you are. You have the opportunity, now, to really enjoy the comfort of this analgesic. To feel comfortable and at ease. Free from tension and tightness and stress and pain. So very comfortable and at ease.

And of course, any feelings of greater comfort that you create, any ability that you have for imagining the analgesic doing its job, are abilities that you have. And the more you practice, the better you will be. Any feelings and improvements that you are noticing can stay with you, and linger beyond the session. They can last for minutes, hours, days, and even years after you are done. The more you practice, the more they can become a permanent part of what your mind gives to you. As natural as breathing. The benefits from your self-hypnosis are becoming an automatic part of who you are.

And now, if you wish, you can allow your eyes to close and enjoy the state you are in for as long as would like. Taking the time you need to come back to the here and now. When you are ready to come back to the here and now, you can signal to yourself that you are ready by allowing your eyes to open. And when they do, you will be comfortable and alert . . . ready to go on to do whatever it is that you would like to do next.

And now, allow your whole body to relax. Allow all your muscles to go limp. Give yourself some time, right now, to notice how all of your muscles are relaxing . . .

And then allow special muscle groups to relax even more. Starting with the right hand. Imagine that all the muscles and tendons in the right hand are relaxing. And as it relaxes, notice any sensations that let you know that the hand feels more relaxed. Perhaps a sense of warmth, or heaviness, an interesting tingling sensation. Limp, heavy, warm, and comfortable.

And when you notice that the right hand *is* relaxed, allow that relaxation to spread. Up into the wrist, forearm, elbow, and upper arm. The whole right arm becoming more and more relaxed, relaxed and heavy. All the tension draining away, as the arm feels heavier, and heavier, almost as if it were made of lead. So comfortable, so relaxed.

Now allow your awareness to move to the left hand. Imagine how the left hand is becoming limp, heavy, and relaxed. More and more relaxed, heavier and heavier. All the tension draining away. Letting yourself be aware of any sensation that lets you know that the left hand is relaxing, a warmth, a heaviness, any sensation that lets you know that the left hand is becoming more and more relaxed. And then allowing the relaxation to spread. Up the wrist, forearm, through the elbow, and into the upper arm. So very relaxed, heavy, and comfortable.

And as this process continues, as you continue to allow both arms to feel more and more relaxed, you can be aware that the relaxation continues to spread, into the shoulders. All the muscles in the shoulders letting go, relaxing. Letting all the tension drain out of the shoulders.

And the relaxation continues to spread, into the neck. All the muscles and tendons of the neck letting go, one by one. Just allowing the head to rest, as you feel more and more comfortable, more and more at ease. The whole body becoming relaxed, heavy, calm, and peaceful.

Allow the relaxation to spread up around the ears, scalp, letting all the tension drain away. The muscles around the eyes letting go, as do the muscles in the jaw, limp, relaxed, comfortable, and at peace. As relaxed as you have ever been.

And the relaxation continues, down the back. Into your chest. The stomach. And pelvis.

And then down into the legs. First, the right leg, feeling so very heavy, and comfortable. Limp, heavy, and comfortable. Feeling the support of the chair, as the right leg is feeling heavier, heavier, and heavier, and so comfortable. And then the left leg. All the tension draining out of the left leg, to be replaced by comfort. A heavy, pleasant, comfortable and deep relaxation.

Take as long as you wish, now, to enjoy feeling more relaxed. Knowing that you created these feelings yourself. And if it is helpful for you, any feelings of relaxation that you created today can stay with you, and linger beyond the session. Lasting for minutes, hours, days, and even years after you are done. The more you practice, the more these feelings can become a permanent part of what your mind gives to you. As natural as breathing. The benefits from your self-hypnosis are becoming an automatic part of who you are.

And now, if you wish, you can allow your eyes to close and enjoy the state you are in for as long as you would like. Taking the time you need to come back to the here and now. When you are ready to come back to the here and now, you can signal to yourself that you are ready by allowing your eyes to open. And when they do, you will be comfortable and alert . . . ready to go on to do whatever it is that you would like to do next.

With every breath you take, breathing comfort in and breathing discomfort out, you can enjoy the comfort you have created for yourself. You may be pleased, of course, but you may also be surprised that it's so much easier now to simply not notice uncomfortable feelings, to simply not pay attention to anything other than your comfort. So much easier to enjoy the relaxing, peaceful comfort of each breath. So simple, so natural, to attend to your breathing.

And you can also consider how pleased and surprised you might be to notice that, as your mind is more and more able to eliminate or reduce any uncomfortable sensations, even before you become aware of them, that . . . *you are experiencing fewer and fewer pain flare-ups* . . . and those that you might be aware of at times just seem to be less intense . . . and they last for shorter and shorter periods of time. Your mind is now able to identify them and reduce them. Those sensations that used to be uncomfortable are also much, much less bothersome . . . it is almost as if a part of your mind might notice them at some level, but because you know that they provide little useful information, you are able to ignore them . . . and not be bothered by them at all. Isn't it interesting how your mind is become increasingly able to reduce, eliminate, and ignore all of the old uncomfortable sensations?

And this ability of your mind, to reduce and ignore sensations that used to be interpreted as uncomfortable—maybe even before your conscious mind is aware of these sensations—this ability, this skill, is improving every time you practice. And the more you practice, the more able your mind will be to exert this skill, a skill that you continue to develop, more and more.

So relaxed, so comfortable, yet so interested to see yourself become more skilled, and more able to reduce the frequency, intensity, and duration of any pain flare-ups. So skilled, in fact, that you may be surprised just how infrequently they do occur, if at all. You are becoming so able to manage these, in fact, that they are hardly a problem at all, perhaps even not a problem at all.

Take as long as you wish, now, to enjoy any feelings of confidence, relaxation, and comfort. Knowing that you created these feelings yourself. And if it is helpful for you, any of these feelings that you created today can stay with you, and linger beyond the session. Lasting for minutes, hours, days, and even years after you are done. The more you practice, the more these feelings can become a permanent part of what your mind gives to you.

As natural as breathing. The benefits from your self-hypnosis are becoming an automatic part of who you are.

And now, if you wish, you can allow your eyes to close and enjoy the state you are in for as long as would like. Taking the time you need to come back to the here and now. When you are ready to come back to the here and now, you can signal to yourself that you are ready by allowing your eyes to open. And when they do, you will be comfortable and alert . . . ready to go on to do whatever it is that you would like to do next.

And you can take a moment, now, to remember that the natural state of the body is to feel energized after periods of rest. Your body and mind will let you know when it is a good time to rest. And then after you rest, to feel energized again. The natural pattern and rhythm of our lives is to rest, feel energized, rest, and feel energized. Back and forth. You know this well. It is how your mind and body has worked since even before you were born.

What might be useful to also remember—and you may find this very useful indeed—is that you can allow yourself periods of rest when it is appropriate. You can use brief self-hypnosis to give your mind and body the rest it needs, so that you can feel energized throughout the day. After periods of rest, you can really experience a sense of energy. A sense of being able to accomplish what it is you want to accomplish.

In fact, you have already been resting for a number of minutes today. Just now, as you practice self-hypnosis. So that you can know that when you are done with this session, you can wake up and feel rested and energized. Just feel good.

And then, when it is time for you take a brief rest, you can allow yourself to do. It need not be a long rest. Just enough to let your body and mind pull together the resources to feel energetic again. Maybe 5 minutes, maybe even just 1 minute.

You can find a comfortable place. Take a nice deep breath and hold it . . . hold it . . . and let it go. Allow the eyes to close and just let your mind and body . . . *rest*. And when you wake up, you will feel rested and energized.

Fatigue becomes a thing of the past. When you need to feel more energy, you can take a nice, brief, self-hypnotic rest. It might be twice a day on some days. It might be every hour on other days. You know what is best for you. And you can pace yourself with periods of rest followed by periods of feeling so energetic. So that when you are awake, you feel energized, alert, focused. And the periods of rest, when you use them, can feel so restful, relaxing.

All of the time, every day, throughout the day, you feel good. Sometimes relaxed, in a nice restful self-hypnosis state. Sometimes energized, doing what is important and meaningful.

Take as long as you wish, now, to enjoy any feelings of relaxation, rest, and energy that you created for yourself. And if it is helpful for you, know that any of the feelings that you created today can stay with you, and linger beyond the session. Lasting for minutes, hours, days, and even years after you are done. The more you practice, the more these feelings can become a permanent part of what your mind gives to you. As natural as breathing. The benefits from your self-hypnosis are becoming an automatic part of who you are.

And now, if you wish, you can allow your eyes to close and enjoy the state you are in for as long as would like. Taking the time you need to come back to the here and now. When you are ready to come back to the here and now, you can signal to yourself that you are ready by allowing your eyes to open. And when they do, you will be rested, alert, and energized . . . ready to go on to do whatever it is that you would like to do next.

Response to Self-Hypnosis Form

Date: _____ Induction used: _____ Suggestion used: _____

Overall, my response to the self-hypnosis session was:

( ) Very positive; I felt much better during and after the session

( ) Somewhat positive; I felt somewhat better during and after the session

( ) Neutral; I did not notice any changes in how I felt during or after the session

( ) Somewhat negative; I felt worse during and after the session

( ) Very negative; I felt much worse during and after the session

What changed for you during or after the session?

_____

_____

_____

_____

The components of the session that seemed most helpful were (list each one):

_____

_____

_____

_____

_____

The components of the session that seemed less helpful were (list each one):

_____

_____

_____

_____

_____

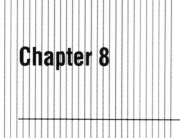

Chapter 8

Using Self-Hypnosis for Thought and Mood Management

Goal

- To learn and practice three hypnotic suggestions for thought and mood management

Chapter Overview

You know from what you read in Chapter 2 of this workbook that your thoughts can have a profound influence on your mood, which in turn affects how you experience pain. This chapter presents three suggestions that you can use to focus your mind on adaptive and reassuring thoughts, so that you experience less pain and feel a greater sense of well-being. The first suggestion, one for tolerating ambiguity, provides an important foundation for being able to shift more easily from unhelpful to helpful thoughts. The second suggestion is designed to increase the frequency with which you think helpful and reassuring thoughts. The final suggestion uses "time projection," a strategy to help you identify creative new thoughts that will help you make the changes you wish for.

Tolerating Ambiguity

Michael Yapko, PhD, a prominent clinician and teacher in the field, has emphasized the importance of being able to tolerate ambiguity in order to feel more comfortable and avoid anxiety and other negative feelings. He points out in his writings that often people with anxiety and depression fall into the trap of automatically jumping to conclusions about events and situations in their lives. This would be fine if the conclusions had no effects on people's mood or pain.

The fact is, though, that the conclusions people make about themselves and the events in their lives have significant and important consequences. When those conclusions are unhelpful and alarming (for example, thinking "My pain stops me from being able to go to the movies with my friends" or "I *must* reduce the pain before I can think about anything else"), they feel bad. Also, because of the way the brain works, they can also experience higher levels of pain.

A first step to sorting helpful from unhelpful thoughts is to give yourself permission to pause; there is no need to draw conclusions about your pain or other issues in your life too soon. To accomplish this, you need to be able to tolerate ambiguity—to allow yourself to "not know" about the future, or to "not know" why an event happened. If you feel that you "must know," then there is a risk that you will conclude something that is both incorrect and unhelpful.

For example, imagine that your spouse and teenager are late for dinner and attempts to reach them by phone have been unsuccessful. You could immediately draw all kinds of conclusions about this event: "They've been in a terrible accident," or "They're doing this just to annoy me," or "The police stopped them because they were speeding again." Although it is possible that one of these scenarios explains their absence, the fact is that you do not know why they are late. Importantly, thinking these alarming thoughts will likely make you feel frightened, angry, or frustrated.

An alternative is to hold off on making any judgments or conclusions, to tolerate not knowing what happened. You could think, "I don't know why they're late. Maybe they were held up in traffic. Maybe they stopped to help someone in trouble. I really don't know for sure." Such "not knowing" thoughts tend to be more helpful because they allow for the possibility of thoughts that might help you to feel more reassured and calm.

The goal of the suggestion on pages 116–117 is to increase your ability to tolerate ambiguity and to feel more comfortable "not knowing" the reasons for what happens to you and around you. The more comfortable you are with ambiguity, the more time you have to monitor and evaluate the many possible reasons for the events that occur, and perhaps select the reason that is most accurate and also that gives you the greatest sense of comfort.

One very effective strategy for training yourself to have helpful thoughts is to specifically identify the thoughts and conclusions that *you* think are reassuring, and then use self-hypnosis to help make these thoughts automatic. You may already have identified such thoughts in treatment sessions with your clinician. You can use self-hypnosis to make these helpful thoughts become the first ones that come to mind, and you can feel better as a result. For this to occur, it is important that (1) the thoughts are helpful and (2) you can endorse them wholeheartedly—in other words, you believe that they are true.

Some potentially helpful thoughts are listed on the Helpful Thoughts Form on page 112. It would be useful to make a photocopy of the form and complete it. The form asks you to identify all of the thoughts that you believe would be helpful, given your current situation, and then to identify the single thought that you believe would be *most* helpful to you. You should bring the completed form with you to your next treatment session, and discuss with your clinician how the wording of this thought might be improved to make it even more helpful, or if another idea or thought not on the Helpful Thoughts Form might be even more useful.

Helpful Thoughts Form

Instructions: A number of thoughts that many individuals with chronic pain find helpful and reassuring are listed below. Please read each thought carefully and decide if you believe that that thought would be helpful and reassuring for *you* to focus on, given your situation. After you read each of the thoughts, go back and select the one thought that you believe would be *most* helpful for you to focus on at this point in time.

Most Helpful?	Helpful?	
( )	( )	No matter what else is happening, it is possible for me to live a life that is in accord with my values.
( )	( )	Pain will never stop me from doing what I really want to do.
( )	( )	I have the skills and resources I need to influence the amount of pain I feel, and the effects that pain has on my life.
( )	( )	I am able to pace my activities so that I can get done what I really want to get done.
( )	( )	Pain will come and pain will go, but I will always be me.
( )	( )	I have the skills to be able to feel relaxed and comfortable whenever I wish.
( )	( )	I can envision a future where I am going to feel even better than I do now.
( )	( )	I have control over how I feel today, how I will feel tomorrow, and beyond.
( )	( )	I have clear goals that I am working towards that will make my life better.
( )	( )	There are people whom I respect who love me and respect me for who I am.
( )	( )	I can have hope for a cure, but I do not need to find a cure for my pain in order to live a life consistent with my most deeply held values.
( )	( )	My brain is capable of *automatically* interrupting any unhelpful thoughts, and then focusing on thoughts that are reassuring and comforting.
( )	( )	I understand from my doctor what activities are safe for me to do, and I have the confidence to be able to do these activities no matter how much pain I might feel.
( )	( )	I am able to manage my pain and my life without medications.
( )	( )	Although I can seek out and experience support from those I am close to, I am able to do what I need to do without help from others.

Once you identify the thought that you believe will be most helpful, make a photocopy of the suggestions presented on pages 118–119, and write that thought in the blank portions of this script. Then you can proceed to induce a hypnotic state via your preferred induction, and read the suggestion. One thing you might notice when you do this is the difference in how you respond to these thought-focusing suggestions compared to your response to the decreased pain and fatigue suggestions presented in the previous chapter. Although everyone's responses to all of these scripts are unique, many patients experience fairly rapid changes in response to the symptom suggestions. However, the changes are often more subtle as you shift your thinking to helpful and reassuring thoughts. You will more likely find yourself feeling better hours after self-hypnosis sessions that focus on thoughts, rather than necessarily during or immediately after the session. It is as if the benefits of the helpful thoughts take some time to resonate throughout your brain.

In addition to taking the 5 to 10 minutes to engage in a self-hypnotic induction and read the suggestions on pages 118–119, you may want to consider taking the helpful thought that you identified, writing it onto several pieces of paper, and taping those pieces of paper around your house in places you see regularly—on the bathroom mirror, at the bottom of your television screen, and on the refrigerator door. Then, each time that you see the thought, take a brief moment to enter a light hypnotic state (by taking a deep breath, holding it, and letting it go), and then repeat the idea or thought in your mind several times while experiencing the *truth* of the thought. The more that you focus on the helpful thought and repeat it, especially if you do so following a hypnotic induction, the more helpful the thought will be for you.

Using Time Progression to Identify New Reassuring Thoughts and Skills

There are many thoughts and ideas that would likely be helpful to you but that you have not yet identified. The script presented on pages 120–121 is designed to help you find and articulate these thoughts, while also giving you hope about your future. It uses "time progression" suggestions where you imagine yourself at some point in the future when you are doing even better than you are now. The suggestion is based on the work of Moshe Torem, MD, a prominent clinician and writer in the field, who has proposed this strategy as a means of helping individuals with depression. His technique was adapted here to focus on adaptive pain management.

Chapter Summary

The thoughts and ideas that you have about your pain play a significant role in your mood and overall life quality. They can also influence how much you focus on and experience pain. The three suggestions presented in this chapter are designed to help you make a shift from unhelpful to helpful thoughts and ideas. Each of the suggestions does this in a different way. The first suggestion, based in large part on the work of Michael Yapko, PhD, focuses on encouraging you to be able to tolerate ambiguity. This should inhibit any tendencies to "jump to conclusions" about ambiguous events, giving your mind time to consider a number of explanations and ideas about those events, and to select one that is most helpful and reassuring.

The second suggestion is designed to increase the frequency with which you focus on a specific thought that you have identified as being reassuring and useful for you at this point in time. The more you ponder this thought, especially when you are in the receptive state that follows a hypnotic induction, the more you will benefit from its reassuring and calming effects. The final suggestion is designed to let your imagination identify the thoughts and ideas brought back from a version of you who is doing very well "at some time in the future." By letting these creative ideas become a part of your current self, you may identify new ways to feel better now (and not have to wait for the future to benefit).

Suggestions for Tolerating Ambiguity begins on the next page

You know that there are thoughts that you have about yourself and your life that help you to feel at ease and comfortable. You may be discovering more of these thoughts, and practicing focusing on them, feeling better and more optimistic all of the time.

You are also learning to pay attention to your thoughts, and to decide for yourself which ones are more helpful and which ones are less helpful to you—to determine if a thought, idea, or conclusion is reassuring and brings you comfort and confidence.

But of course, it takes *time* to evaluate thoughts—time to let your mind evaluate and then select the thoughts and ideas that are *most* helpful and *most* reassuring.

An important skill to have in this process is to be able to give yourself the time you need to evaluate thoughts and draw conclusions that are most helpful to you. It is a skill to be *open* to many possibilities, *open* to a variety of conclusions, thoughts, and ideas.

For example, imagine that you are at a party, and you see an old friend. As you walk towards the friend, he or she seems to see you, frowns, and walks away. The natural reaction to an event like this might be to wonder, "Why did my friend frown and turn away?" We are all scientists, wondering, asking questions, discovering, and then reaping the rewards of our knowledge, based on a careful evaluation of the evidence.

But in the desire to know and understand, there is also risk, a risk that we will draw the wrong conclusions too quickly—conclusions that may not always be correct or helpful. When asking ourselves, "Why did my friend turn away?" we might come up with potential answers that might not only make us feel bad, but may also simply not be true.

An important skill is to be able to *wait* before drawing final conclusions and to understand that the ideas that can come to us are often just that—ideas. They might be right, they might be wrong. It is a skill to be able to feel comfortable tolerating not knowing, not being sure, until you learn more.

And it is perfectly okay not to know for sure. No one expects you to know everything. No one expects you to be able to predict the future with certainty. It really is the best and brightest scientists who are able to say, "I don't know for sure."

So before you come to a conclusion, you can ask yourself, "Is this conclusion helpful for me? Does it allow me to feel more relaxed, at ease, comfortable, and confident?" If so, you may choose to let that conclusion be an option—one of many. It does not have to be your final conclusion, but it certainly may be worth entertaining, considering, and focusing on.

If the conclusion is less than helpful, you might decide to just table that conclusion for now—to let it go until you obtain more information.

So each and every time you experience an event or situation that can have multiple interpretations, you can remind yourself that there are many ways to think about what happens to you. No two people look at the same event the same way. You can let yourself *not know* the reasons something happened, but consider a variety of interpretations and conclusions. And the more possible interpretations you can come up with, the more options your mind will have for selecting the interpretations that might be most useful to consider and focus on. You can give yourself the time this takes by being comfortable, really comfortable, with not knowing for sure.

You have been using your hypnotic skills for a number of weeks now, and every time you practice you learn something new. Of course, learning never stops; it happens automatically. But it can also be directed in ways that are beneficial to you.

When we first learn something, we often need to really think about it, to focus our attention on what we need to do. Like practicing scales, or practicing a sport, or practicing anything. As we practice, we can enjoy noticing that we are getting better and better and better. And then, all of the sudden, we find we can do something without having to think about it at all. Like riding a bike, or driving, or walking. It happens automatically, freeing up our mind to do something else: have a conversation with someone we enjoy, or listen to the radio. And all it takes is practice. The more we do something, the more automatic it becomes.

And you already know that the ways of thinking about the events in your life can have a profound influence on the way that you feel about yourself, your life, and your future. You can have reassuring, reasonable, and realistic thoughts about events and your symptoms. And these thoughts can bring you comfort and confidence and hope. Part of growing up and becoming more mature and wise is knowing when beliefs are reasonable and reassuring, to be able to form such thoughts and communicate them to yourself and to others.

In fact, you have already identified at least one very clear thought that is just right for you, right here and right now—a thought that brings you comfort. It is the idea that

_____

_____

And to the extent that this thought makes sense and is helpful, you can allow it to sink in. And it can stay with you for as long, *and only as long,* as it *continues to be beneficial to you.* Reassuring you, as if you had a wise and trusted friend in the background, reminding you and reassuring you. So that you notice that you are feeling better and better. Now take a moment to really ponder what this thought means to you . . . take whatever time you need.

And *all* the skills that you have developed in your lifetime, through practice and concentration, these are skills that are now automatic. The brain is doing many things for us automatically: deciding what to focus on, determining when to eat, regulating the body temperature. And regulating your thoughts—by encouraging the mind to monitor all thoughts about any pain or symptoms BEFORE those thoughts reach your consciousness, determining if the thoughts are reasonable and reassuring, and then allowing those thoughts that are most helpful, reassuring, and realistic to come into your consciousness, so that you can feel reassured. And any preliminary ideas that the mind considers as alarming, exaggerated, or unhelpful, those ideas can just fade back into the background, or automatically be modified into ideas and thoughts that are more realistic and reasonable—and *then* be allowed to come into your awareness.

And now, if you wish, you can allow your eyes to close and enjoy the state you are in for as long as would like. Taking the time you need to come back to the here and now. When you are ready to come back to the here and now, you can signal to yourself that you are ready by allowing your eyes to open. And when they do, you will be rested, alert, and energized . . . ready to go on to do whatever it is that you would like to do next.

And now imagine that you are able to travel into your future. You might imagine going through a tunnel of time, or experience yourself stepping into a special time machine. You move into your future when you are managing even better than you are now. I do not know when that will be—it might be a year from now, two years, five, or even 10 years from now. But you are moving forward in time, and then stopping at some point of time when you are doing well, very, very well.

You have successfully learned the cognitive and hypnosis skills you are practicing right now. Your mind is able to note your thoughts and evaluate them quickly, easy, and automatically, and adjust them for you as needed so you can feel more comfortable, physically and emotionally. You are able, whenever you wish, to enter a state of total relaxation, and to calmly evaluate your symptoms so that they do not bother you at all. You can see yourself in your mind's eye feeling so good, actually see yourself, so relaxed, able to manage any symptoms comfortably and easily. Any symptoms really do not bother you. The part of you that is *YOU* is able to focus on and enjoy the things that really matter.

You are no longer surprised at your abilities to manage your thoughts and symptoms. Your skills in this area are now second nature. You see yourself as confident; you can actually see yourself smiling, feeling so good, relaxed, happy, calm, and strong.

And now, as you see your future self, you can experience yourself moving *into* that body. You *become* yourself in the future. You can feel, actually feel, what it is like to feel so good, so confident. Before, you saw yourself smiling. *Now* you can feel yourself smiling. So relaxed. So strong. And in control. You are feeling even better than you imagined you might. You have the abilities and the skills to manage your thoughts and your sensations.

And as you experience being this future you, that feels so good. What is it that you are thinking to yourself or about yourself that allows to you feel this relaxed, calm, and comfortable? Take a few minutes, right now, to pay attention to these thoughts, and note the ones that you think are particularly true and helpful. . .

And now, you can get ready to travel back from the future. Perhaps walking back in the tunnel, or stepping again in your time machine. As you come back, bring with you all of these positive experiences of joy, comfort, delight, accomplishments, skills . . . and *thoughts*. Bring them back as your gifts, gifts from your future self. Allow them to stay with you;

they are *now* a part of you, *now, today*. You have arrived to the present, enjoying and noticing how you are still *you*, but also changed.

These gifts are now really a part of you. New skills and thoughts that are a part of you now, in the present. And they can stay with you. You can carry them into the future over time so that they will be with you, when you are actually living in the future. They will have been with you for all of this time. Now a permanent part of how your mind works. Isn't it interesting how you are using these skills and thoughts, and your ability to imagine, to make a positive difference in your life right now, today . . . and every day?

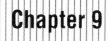
Using Self-Hypnosis for Activity and Sleep Management

Goals

- To learn and practice a hypnotic suggestion for increasing your activity

- To understand the effects of lifestyle habits on your sleep quality

- To learn three simple self-hypnotic strategies for getting to sleep at night

- To learn and practice a hypnotic suggestion for improved sleep

Chapter Overview

The focus of this chapter is on the use of self-hypnosis for helping you change what you *do* to cope with pain, and for improving your sleep. It begins with a hypnotic suggestion that can make it easier to change how you cope with pain, if this is what you decide to do. The next section describes some basic lifestyle habits that influence sleep; putting aside habits that interfere with sleep and practicing habits that improve sleep (called "sleep hygiene") can help you get better sleep at night. The chapter then introduces three simple self-hypnotic strategies for getting to sleep, plus a hypnotic suggestion you can read during self-hypnosis to improve your sleep quality.

Increasing Helpful and Adaptive Pain Coping Responses

You already know, based on what you read in Chapter 2, that how you cope with pain plays an important role in the overall quality of your life and the amount of pain you will experience over time. Resting too much, by far the most common unhelpful pain coping response, will contribute to muscle, tendon, and bone atrophy, making you weaker and increasing the chances that you will experience higher levels of pain in the long run. But there are a number of other unhelpful coping responses that tend to worsen pain over time. Unfortunately, many of these unhelpful efforts at coping result in a temporary decrease in pain in the short run, which can make it difficult to give them up.

One of the goals of most pain treatment programs is to *reduce* the frequency of those behaviors or coping responses that make pain worse in the long run. In pain treatment programs people also learn pain coping responses that can decrease pain and disability in the long run (for example, how to exercise, and how to maintain activities and hobbies that give your life the most meaning). It is important to remember when selecting behavioral goals, however, that what is helpful and unhelpful for one person may or may not be helpful or unhelpful for another person. You should work closely with your clinician and healthcare providers to identify the behavioral goals that are most appropriate for you. In particular, although participating in a regular exercise program is almost always indicated as a way to better manage pain, the specific exercises that are safe and appropriate for you should be identified by your doctor or healthcare provider. Once these are identified, *then* you can develop a plan to integrate those exercises into your life.

The script presented on page 135 is designed to make it easy for you to picture yourself engaging in the behavioral goal that you have identified for yourself. You should make a copy of the script, and then write into each blank space the specific behavioral goal. If, for example, your goal is to increase your endurance so that you could walk a mile every day, you could write in "walk a mile every day" in

And now imagine that you are able to travel into your future. You might imagine going through a tunnel of time, or experience yourself stepping into a special time machine. You move into a future when you are managing even better than you are now. I do not know when that will be—it might be a year from now, two years, five, or even 10 years from now. But you are moving forward in time, and then stopping at some point when you are doing very well, and able to easily *walk a mile every day*.

Take a moment, now, to observe a future version of yourself *walking*. Notice the expression on your face; you may be aware that the future version of you is feeling a little proud, because it is so easy for you to *walk every day*.

And take a moment to become very aware of what is different in your life now that you can *walk for a mile each day*. And then take a moment to think about what is better in your life, in the future, because you can now *walk for a mile*.

And now, as you see your future self, you can experience yourself moving into that body. You become yourself in the future, and you can feel, actually feel, what it is like to be able to *walk for a mile every day*. Take a moment to feel yourself *walking*; actually feel as if you are doing it, right now. Take a moment to really feel this. Enjoy all of the good feelings and benefits that this brings you.

And I wonder, what was it that allowed you to get to this point, to be able *to walk a mile every day* so easily? Think back; how did you achieve this? What did you do? You may want to take a moment to consider this, and then bring this as advice back to your current self.

And now, you can get ready to travel back from the future. Perhaps walking back in the tunnel, or stepping again in your time machine. As you come back, bring with you any of the good feelings you felt while you were *walking*. And bring back, perhaps, a sense of confidence that you are actually able to *walk for a mile every day*, or be able to *walk this much*, at some point in the near future. And finally, you may decide to bring back with you any advice that you would like to give to yourself—advice regarding how you will be able to accomplish this goal.

And now, if you wish, you can allow your eyes to close and enjoy the state you are in for as long as would like. Taking the time you need to come back to the here and now. When you are ready to come back to the here and now, you can signal to yourself that you are ready by allowing your eyes to open. And when they do, you will be rested, alert, and energized . . . ready to go on to do whatever it is that you would like to do next.

Figure 9.1

Sample completed time progression script with helpful coping responses

the first blank space, and then add text at each subsequent blank space as appropriate (see Fig. 9.1 for a sample completed script).

As with all of the other self-hypnosis scripts presented in this workbook, all you need to do is use your favorite self-hypnosis induction, and then sit comfortably in the relaxed hypnotic state and read the script slowly. Give yourself time to respond to each sentence, and experience what the script suggests that you experience. As you repeat this exercise, you will increase your confidence in your ability to engage in the new coping behavior or behavioral goal.

Improved Sleep

Brain Activity during Sleep

One of the many positive "side effects" of hypnosis treatment is improved sleep. To help you to understand why, it is useful to understand how the brain responds as a person sleeps through the night. You may be aware that during a good night's sleep the brain goes through different stages. You do not just "go to sleep" and then remain unconscious for as long as you sleep, only to "wake up" when you are done sleeping.

First, when you are awake, your brain is usually quite active. Your brain cells are firing and talking with each other; back and forth. If someone were to place electrodes on your scalp and record the electrical activity of your brain, they would see a lot of "fast" activity. This activity is associated with a person thinking, doing, and planning. This is the kind of brain activity that goes on when we are awake and going through our day.

As you start to become relaxed before going to sleep, fewer brain cells in the brain are "firing." The brain starts to "calm down" and you start to feel more relaxed. We can see this slowing when we measure the electrical activity in the brain as people are falling asleep. What we see is an increase in "alpha" and "theta" brain waves as a person relaxes. The brain cells are firing more slowly.

From this stage, people usually first drift into a light sleep. Although this is usually the first stage of sleep they enter, it is called "stage 2" sleep. If someone were to wake you up during this stage of sleep, you might say that you did not even feel like you were asleep—that you were just kind of drifting along, not thinking about very much.

Soon, people usually move from stage 2 sleep into a deeper stage of sleep. Even fewer brain cells are active in the next sleep stage; the brain really starts to slow down. Stage 3 sleep is when there is a lot—between 30% and 50%—of very slow brain activity. If you were woken up from stage 3 sleep, you would be somewhat disoriented. You would say that you do not remember much of anything going through your mind.

Once the amount of very slow brain activity reaches 50% or more, the person has entered the deepest stage of sleep, stage 4 sleep. People can be difficult to wake from stage 4 sleep, and when they do wake up, they can be *very* disoriented. They may not know where they are for a moment.

After spending some time in stage 4 sleep, the brain starts to become active again. It moves into stage 3 sleep, and then into stage 2 sleep. And then it does something very interesting. The very fast brain activity returns—the brain looks like it is very active. In fact, it looks a lot like the person is awake, and yet the person is clearly asleep. Also, the eyes start to move around, almost as if they are looking at objects or tracking movement. This is called stage 1-rapid eye movement (or stage 1-REM) sleep. People who wake up during this stage of sleep usually report that they were dreaming.

After spending some time in this stage, the whole cycle starts over again. Sometimes people wake up briefly at this stage just after they dream. Pretty soon, though, they slip back down into stage 2, then into stage 3, and into stage 4 sleep. Then they come back up again.

Each cycle lasts about 90 minutes. And as the night progresses, people tend to spend less time in the deeper stages of sleep (stages 3 and 4) and more time in the lighter stages of sleep (stages 1-REM and 2).

Each stage of sleep seems to be important to our health and well-being. If you deprive people of stage 4 sleep, for example, by waking them up every time they enter stage 4 sleep, they will report that they feel very sleepy during the day. Also, when they are later allowed to sleep without being woken up, they will spend more time in stage 4 sleep than usual, as if they are trying to catch up on the stage 4 sleep they missed. When people get the stage 4 sleep that they need, they report that they feel rested when they wake up.

Likewise, if you wake up a person every time he or she starts to get stage 1-REM sleep, so that he or she isn't allowed to get much of this sleep stage, the person usually reports that he or she feels more anxious and upset during the day—as if this stage of sleep allows him or her to feel more calm. When the person is later allowed to sleep uninterrupted, he or she will then spend more time in this stage of sleep than usual, again as if he or she is trying to catch up on the stage 1-REM sleep that was missed.

People need different amounts of sleep, and they usually know what their ideal amount of sleep is. Saying that everyone needs 7 to 8 hours of sleep every night is like saying that everyone should wear a size medium shirt. Also, our need for sleep seems to decrease a little as we get older. A baby sleeps many more hours than a teenager. Teenagers need more sleep than adults, and young adults need more sleep than older adults. So if you are finding that you are sleeping less as you get older, that is not necessarily a problem. Waking up at night is also not necessarily a problem; we all start to wake up more at night as we get older. The important thing is to be able to get back to sleep when you do wake up so that you feel rested in the morning.

It is also important to understand that your sleep depends on the activity in your brain. And here's what's interesting: you can control the activity in your brain using the self-hypnosis skills that you have been learning. During hypnosis, and in response to hypnotic inductions, the brain starts to slow down, much like it does just before a person falls asleep. We see an increase in alpha and theta brain waves during this transition period. During hypnosis, the brain is *not* asleep; it is just in a state very similar to that stage prior to falling asleep. This means, though, that *you can use your self-hypnosis skills to help you get to sleep at night*, and to get back to sleep if you wake up in the middle of the night. The section later in the chapter entitled "Nighttime Self-Hypnosis Strategies for Getting to Sleep and Getting Back to Sleep" explains how you can do this.

Sleep Hygiene

Sleep hygiene refers to lifestyle behaviors that can influence sleep quality. There are many things that people can do *during the day*, before they even go to sleep, that can make it easier or more difficult to get a good night's sleep. If your pain is making it difficult to get to sleep or stay asleep, you should know about sleep hygiene in case you happen to be doing the things that can interfere with sleeping at night, or not doing the things that can make sleep easier.

Some people are able to sleep whenever they need to. When it is time for them to get to sleep, they go to bed, lie down on their pillow, and fall asleep within minutes. They sleep through the night and wake up feeling rested and refreshed. Part of what may help these people sleep so well is that they have developed good sleep hygiene habits. These good sleep habits fall into three categories: (1) getting your body ready for sleep, (2) getting your mind ready for sleep, and (3) getting your bedroom ready for sleep.

Getting Your Body Ready for Sleep

In order to sleep well, the body should be free of chemicals that can interfere with sleep. This includes all stimulants (caffeine and nicotine) as well as alcohol. The reason to avoid stimulants is probably self-evident: because they can keep your mind active and awake. People who are having a hard time sleeping should avoid beverages containing caffeine (including black tea, many soda drinks, and coffee) at least six hours before bedtime. People who are having a very difficult time with sleep may want to avoid caffeine altogether. If you smoke, avoid smoking in the evening and also anytime at night if you wake up, because nicotine is another stimulant that can interfere with sleep.

Alcohol can help you get to sleep, but it also often causes you to wake up during the night. Even if you sleep through the night after drinking alcohol, alcohol still interferes with your getting the type of sleep that you need, and so you will often end up not feeling rested. Therefore, if you feel tired during the day, or feel that you are not getting good sleep at night, it is best to avoid alcohol.

You should also avoid taking naps during the day if you have trouble sleeping at night (naps during the day are fine if you are able to get restful sleep during the night). If you sleep during the day, your body will feel less need to sleep at night. Regular exercise is good for sleep, as long as you do not do it too close to bedtime.

It is also very useful to get your body in a natural rhythm by waking up at about the same time every day, even on weekends. Over time, and depending on how much sleep you really need, you will start to feel sleepy at about the same time every night, and should plan on going to bed at about that time. Keeping with the same schedule will allow your body to find its rhythm.

Finally, you should avoid eating a heavy meal before going to sleep, as this too can interfere with the sleep cycle. If you are hungry, then having a small snack such as a small glass of milk and a cracker or a piece of fruit might be okay.

Getting Your Mind Ready for Sleep

To help you slip automatically and easily to sleep when you go to bed, it is best to prepare your mind for sleep. You may be aware that the mind automatically links certain reactions to specific events and even specific times. If you see someone you like, you will automatically and immediately feel glad to see him or her, without even having to think about it. People who have been bitten by a dog might automatically feel frightened or at least a little uneasy if they see a dog like the one that bit them.

You can take advantage of this ability of your mind to link events and actions to automatic responses. The idea is to associate certain behaviors with getting to sleep. Ideally, you should develop a pre-sleep ritual that you do every night just before going to sleep. It might involve checking all of the locks in your house, followed by brushing your teeth, ending with some light reading or television watching just before going to bed. If you read or watch TV as part of your pre-sleep ritual, you should not do this while in bed. After your pre-sleep ritual, go right to bed. If you follow the same ritual every night, the ritual itself will cue your mind to shift from waking to pre-sleep activity. Then, when you get into bed, you can start your sleep self-hypnosis strategies (discussed in the next section). You should use the bed only for sex or for sleep. Avoid eating, watching television, reading, or discussing important business with your spouse in bed. You want your mind to associate the bed with sleep.

If you do not fall asleep within 15 or 20 minutes of going to bed, get out of bed. Do something else, perhaps some reading or other non-stimulating activity, until you get sleepy again. You do not want to associate the bed with trying unsuccessfully to get to sleep; you want to associate the bed with sleep. Then, when you get sleepy again, you can go back to bed.

Getting Your Bedroom Ready for Sleep

Make sure that your bed is comfortable. Avoid waterbeds. In general, people sleep better on firmer mattresses than they do on soft ones. People also tend to sleep better in a cool room with thick blankets than they do in a warm room with thin blankets. Also, of course, common sense would suggest that you should block out any sources of light and noise. If you live in a noisy area, you might find that a white noise (or ocean sound) generator helps. Finally, if you are a "clock watcher," it is best to eliminate the temptation to keep looking at your clock by facing it toward the wall.

Nighttime Self-Hypnosis Strategies for Getting to Sleep and Getting Back to Sleep

If you are having a difficult time getting or staying asleep, then following the sleep hygiene recommendations just described should allow to you get to sleep faster, stay asleep longer, and feel more rested when you wake up in the morning. In addition, you can use your self-hypnosis skills for getting to sleep.

For example, you can use your favorite hypnotic induction just as you are planning to get to sleep. It could be any of the three inductions you learned in Chapter 6 of this workbook. Or it might be an induction that you learned in your work with your clinician. Virtually anytime you focus your awareness on a stimulus or image, the brain's response is to decrease fast-wave (beta) activity and increase slow-wave (alpha and theta) activity. There is less "chatter" in the mind; you are too busy noticing the details of your safe place or experiencing feelings of relaxation to worry and ruminate. From this state, if the brain and body need sleep, you will more easily slip into sleep.

For some people (but not all people, so don't worry if you don't have this response), a natural muscular response to relaxation is to "twitch." So if you notice that different muscles twitch slightly, you can take it as a good sign; a sign that you are relaxing. It this case, you might find it interesting to count the twitches as they occur. If you do, you will also notice that fairly soon you will lose track of the number of twitches, or even forget to count altogether. This inability to count and keep track is another sign that your brain is drifting into the first stages of sleep.

A second experience sometimes associated with drifting off to sleep is that of random visual images—either "dreamlike" images of objects or people, or simply colors and patterns. If you are a person who experiences these images, your job is to simply notice and enjoy them as they occur, and to understand that they are a sign that you are getting control over the process of getting to sleep. When you wake up in the middle of the night—and most adults, in particular older adults, do—you can simply use your favorite hypnotic induction to get your mind into a state where it is easy to get to sleep again.

An excellent self-hypnosis induction that some people enjoy is called the "3-2-1" technique. I first heard about this technique from a colleague and clinician named Björn Enqvist. The goal of the 3-2-1 technique is the same as the other self-hypnotic inductions: it gives you something interesting to focus your attention on and experience as your mind slows down.

The 3-2-1 technique is very simple. First, just *listen* for three things. Any three things that you hear as you are going to sleep will do: the noise of your breathing—one; or maybe a sound of a far-off airplane—two; or maybe the sound of your skin against the sheet— three. Any three things at all. They can even be the same thing. Just listen for, hear, and then count three things.

Next, *feel* three things; any three things. For example, the feeling of the sheet against your skin—one; an interesting tingling sensation in your arms—two; and cool or maybe warm air on your face—three. It does not matter what they are. Any three things will do. They can be different or the same. Just feel them and count them, 1, 2, 3.

And then, *see* three things. Allow three images to come into the mind. Just let them appear, on their own. A rose—one. A blue sky— two. Some third image; it does not matter what it is, maybe a beach—three. Any three images.

Then, after you have seen the third thing, go back and hear *two* things, and count them in the mind. Then feel two things. Then see two things. Then hear one thing, feel one thing, and see one thing.

And then start again. Hear three things, feel three things, see three things. Then hear two things, feel two things, see two things. Then hear, feel, and see one thing. And back to three.

As the mind focuses on and is experiencing what it hears, feels, and sees, and as it starts to drift to sleep, you will likely lose count. That is fine; just start over. Hear, feel, and see three things. Hear, feel, and see two things. Hear, feel, and see one thing. You can use this strategy and discover what interesting things you can experience as you drift into a deep, restful sleep.

Daytime Self-Hypnosis Suggestions for Improved Sleep

In addition to using your self-hypnotic inductions or the 3-2-1 technique at night, you may also choose to read the hypnotic suggestions presented on pages 136–137 during the day to enhance the efficacy of your self-hypnosis. These suggestions can be incorporated into your self-hypnosis practice after the usual self-guided induction.

Chapter Summary

Pain can have a significant and negative impact on many aspects of a person's life, including the ability to do what is most meaningful and important, and the ability to get restful sleep. What you do to cope with your pain influences how much pain interferes with your life. Thinking about and using adaptive pain coping strategies gives you yet another option for managing your pain, and you can use hypnosis to facilitate this process.

An important first step is to determine, with input from your clinician and healthcare providers, which changes might be needed so that you can ultimately hurt less and do more. Most patients find that some change in their activity level and exercise program is needed. Others may need help reducing or eliminating some medications that are causing more problems than they are solving (although certain medications for some patients can be very helpful; consult with your physician before considering making any changes in your medications). Once you identify a behavioral or lifestyle change that you think will be helpful, you can use hypnosis to make that change easier (see the script for increasing helpful pain coping responses on page 135).

Because sleep problems are so common in persons with chronic pain, it is useful to learn about sleep and what you can do to have restful sleep more often. Knowledge about brain activity during sleep helps you to understand how self-hypnosis, which alters brain activity, is useful. You can also improve your sleep quality by making relatively simple changes in your behavior during the day; for example, by avoiding chemicals that interfere with sleep (caffeine, nicotine, and alcohol), avoiding naps during the day, waking up and getting out of bed at about the same time every day, using the bed only for sex or sleep, and developing a pre-sleep ritual that you engage in on a regular basis. You can use one or more of your favorite self-hypnosis inductions to prepare your mind for sleep at night, or to help you get back to sleep if you wake up. Finally, you can read self-hypnosis suggestions during the day to enhance the efficacy of your self-hypnosis inductions.

As you increase the use of adaptive pain coping behaviors, engage in more activities that are most meaningful to you, and get more restful sleep at night, you should note an overall increase in the quality of your life—pain will have less of a negative impact. A common "side effect" of these changes is also a decrease in pain.

Time Progression Suggestions for Increasing Helpful Pain Coping Responses

And now imagine that you are able to travel into your future. You might imagine going through a tunnel of time, or experience yourself stepping into a special time machine. You move into a future when you are managing even better than you are now. I do not know when that will be—it might be a year from now, two years, five, or even 10 years from now. But you are moving forward in time, and then stopping at some point of time when you are doing very well, and able to easily _____.

Take a moment, now, to observe a future version of yourself _____. Notice the expression on your face; you may be aware that the future you is feeling a little proud, because it is so easy for you to _____.

And take a moment to become very aware of what is different in your life now that you can _____. And then take a moment to think about what is better in your life, in the future, because you can now _____.

And now, as you see your future self, you can experience yourself moving *into* that body. You *become* yourself in the future, and you can feel, actually feel, what it is like to be able to _____. Take a moment, to feel yourself _____; actually feel as if you are doing it, right *now*. Take a moment to really feel this. Enjoy all of the good feelings and benefits that this brings you.

And I wonder, what was it that allowed you to get to this point, to be able to _____ so easily? Think back; how did you achieve this? What did you do? You may want to take a moment to consider this, and then bring this as advice to your current self.

And now, you can get ready to travel back from the future. Perhaps walking back in the tunnel, or stepping again in your time machine. As you come back, bring with you any of the good feelings you felt while you were _____. And bring back, perhaps, a sense of confidence that you are actually able to _____, or be able to _____, at some point in the near future. And finally, you may decide to bring back with you any advice that you would like to give to yourself— advice regarding how you will be able to accomplish this goal.

And now, if you wish, you can allow your eyes to close and enjoy the state you are in for as long as would like. Taking the time you need to come back to the here and now. When you are ready to come back to the here and now, you can signal to yourself that you are ready by allowing your eyes to open. And when they do, you will be rested, alert, and energized . . . ready to go on to do whatever it is that you would like to do next.

You know that the state of relaxation, the state you have reached now, is not sleep. It is a state of focused awareness and an increased ability to alter your brain state. Yet we also know that some parts of the brain are not very active during this state. The brain is relaxed. This state is very much like the state you are in right before you go to sleep.

And you can use your ability to enter the state you are in now to be able to easily slip into a state of sleep later. All you have to do is take a nice deep breath, hold it, hold it for a moment . . . and let it go. And the mind will slow down, relax, become more focused. And if you are ready the mind can slip into a nice, deep, restful sleep. But what will you do as you wait? You have many options . . . as long as they are relaxing and comfortable and interesting.

When it is time for you to get to sleep, you might decide to simply practice one of your inductions—for example, the relaxation induction where you gradually move from one body part to another, imagining each body part feeling more relaxed. A key is to really enjoy the sensations of relaxation that you create for yourself. As you lie there feeling relaxed, and as you are enjoying the relaxing feelings, if your brain and body need sleep, they will drift off into sleep. When you next wake up, and if you need more sleep, you can just repeat the exercise.

Or, you know that as the body and mind relax, muscles twitch. Sometimes they twitch a tiny little bit and sometimes they make larger movements. When it is time to sleep, it can be interesting to allow yourself to pay very, very close attention to the movements and twitches of the body as it becomes more and more relaxed and enters a state of sleep. Each twitch, each movement, means the body is more relaxed. And you can feel yourself relaxing with every one, so that when you are ready to go to sleep at night, you can simply pay attention to and count the twitches. No need to worry if you lose track of the number; just start again and keep counting until you enter a deep, restful sleep.

I do not know which strategy you will find most helpful or use most often. I do not know which one will give you the most sense of control over your mind. Maybe many strategies will work well for you, and you will use different ones on different nights. But I do know that each one can help you to get to sleep whenever you wish. And the sleep you achieve will be restful and comfortable.

And now, if you wish, you can allow your eyes to close and enjoy the state you are in for as long as would like. Taking the time you need to come back to the here and now. When you are ready to come back to the here and now, you can signal to yourself that you are ready by allowing your eyes to open. And when they do, you will be rested, alert, and energized . . . ready to go on to do whatever it is that you would like to do next.

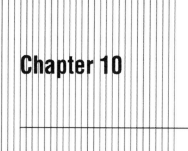

Chapter 10   *Summary and Conclusions*

Goal

■ To review the information presented in this workbook

Chapter Overview

This patient workbook provides you with the basic information you need to be able to use self-hypnosis to help you better manage pain and its effects on your life. It is best read and used when working closely with a clinician who is experienced in the use of hypnosis for pain management. This final chapter provides a summary of the information included in the entire workbook and discusses some additional issues that should be considered as you continue to use your self-hypnosis skills to make your life better.

Workbook Summary

How Your Body and Brain Create Pain

We have learned a great deal about how the body and brain work together to create the experience that is labeled pain. We now know that *all* pain is real, and all pain is created by the brain. We also know that there is no "pain center" in the brain. Rather, it is activity in different areas of the brain and body, all working together, that creates pain sensations.

The parts of the brain that contribute to pain include those areas responsible for the meaning we give to pain (prefrontal cortex), the intensity and quality of pain (sensory cortices), the suffering component of pain (anterior cingulate cortex), and the extent to which we judge that our body is physically at risk (insula). These areas of the brain communicate with each other, so treatments that influence one area will affect activity in the other areas. With training and practice, you can learn to get control over these areas of the brain, and feel less pain.

Thoughts and Coping Influence Pain

What you think about your pain and what you do to cope with pain will affect how much pain you feel, and how it influences your life. The goal of any pain treatment program should be to help you use coping responses that will ultimately allow you to feel better, and to reduce or eliminate any thoughts and coping responses that make you feel worse. What can make this difficult is that the coping responses that help you feel better in the long run may require more effort, and can produce some discomfort at first. Exercise is probably the best example of this. But with self-hypnosis you can more easily make the changes you decide to make in your life and lifestyle.

Based on what scientists have discovered, it is possible to have a fairly clear picture of what a person who is managing well with chronic pain well looks like. Such an individual would rarely, if ever, think alarming and negative thoughts about or in response to pain. He or she would also rarely, if ever, rest in response to pain. When experiencing pain, he or she would probably not ask for help with a chore that he or she is capable of doing. Rather, this person would be thinking realistic, reassuring, and adaptive thoughts—thoughts reflecting a sense of control over pain and its effects—and would use adaptive pain coping responses to manage pain. You should work closely with your primary healthcare provider and clinician to develop a plan for the changes that you want to make in how you think about pain and how you cope with pain, so that over time you can do more and hurt less.

What Is Hypnosis?

Hypnosis can be defined as a procedure in which one person (the subject) is guided by another person (the hypnotist) to respond to suggestions for changes in how the person feels or what he or she does. It usually begins with an induction inviting the subject to focus his or her attention. The induction is associated with changes in brain activity that allow the subject to feel more relaxed and focused.

People are also more open to responding to suggestions after a hypnotic induction. The induction is followed by a suggestion or set of suggestions for experiencing beneficial changes. With *self-hypnosis*, the subject learns to enter a hypnotic state him or herself, using one or more inductions. The subject can then read suggestions from a script, or if those suggestions have been memorized, just repeat the positive suggestions in his or her own mind. Hypnosis can be effectively used to change the amount of pain you experience, what you think about pain, how you cope with pain, or your sleep quality.

Different theories have been proposed to explain the effects of hypnosis, and each one helps us to understand a little more about how hypnosis works. They also help us to understand that there is nothing "magic" or mysterious about hypnosis. Its effects and benefits are very real.

What Hypnosis Can Do for Pain

Scientists have discovered that hypnosis has measurable effects on all of the brain areas and body processes that are involved in the creation of pain. It has been shown to reduce inflammatory responses in the skin, change how messages are processed in the spinal cord, and decrease or disrupt activity in the areas of the brain that create pain. These findings help explain what clinicians who have used hypnosis have known for hundreds of years: the effects of hypnosis on pain are real, and they can be profound.

Most people can learn to use hypnosis and self-hypnosis to feel more relaxed and comfortable whenever they wish. Many of these individuals will find that the improvements in pain last and linger beyond the hypnosis sessions, and result in long-lasting reductions in pain, freeing them up to focus on activities that are important to them. Hypnosis can also help you to fill your mind with reassuring and relaxing thoughts, which can help to reduce pain and the suffering associated with pain even more.

Hypnosis for Chronic Pain Management: The Basics

What some people "know" about hypnosis is often learned from depictions in movies, on television, or on stage. Unfortunately, much of this information is wrong. Hypnosis is not the same as sleep.

It does not give another person "control" over the hypnotic subject. Moreover, response to hypnosis is unrelated to being "weak-minded" or gullible; virtually everyone is capable of entering a relaxed and focused state, and in this state they can use their imagination to help themselves feel better. People do not usually lose conscious awareness during hypnosis, and they do not need to experience a "deep" level of focused attention to benefit. At the same time, they need not remember *everything* that occurred during a hypnosis session to benefit. Finally, clinical hypnosis is not at all like stage hypnosis. With clinical hypnosis, the goal is to help the patient learn to use his or her ability to control brain activity to feel better. Clinical hypnosis seeks to give patients skills that they will find useful for getting control over pain and its effects. The "side effects" of hypnosis, such as improved sleep, more energy, and an increased sense of well-being, can also improve the overall quality of life.

The goal with hypnosis is to help you make changes in the way that your brain processes pain and pain-related thoughts, so that you can feel better all of the time. To facilitate this, you can listen to audio recordings of your hypnosis sessions between treatment sessions and long after treatment is over. In addition, your clinician may recommend that you practice self-hypnosis on your own, without the audio recordings. You can obtain the benefits of self-hypnosis if you practice for just two or three minutes at a time, several times during a day. Depending on your goals, you may choose to practice even longer.

Practicing Self-Hypnosis: Entering the Hypnotic "State"

You can enter a relaxed hypnotic state using any one of many different induction strategies. This state is the natural response to being absorbed in a stimulus (sound, image, sensation) or activity. Three induction strategies were introduced in this workbook. In a simple countdown induction, you slowly count from 1 to 10, taking a deep breath with every number. You allow yourself to feel increasingly relaxed, heavy, and comfortable as you count. Using a relaxation induction, you systematically imagine each body area feeling heavy, relaxed, and comfortable. With the "safe place" induction, you picture yourself somewhere very safe and comfortable, and while you are there, you pay attention to what you see, smell, feel, and hear.

Each of these inductions usually results in your feeling more comfortable, relaxed, and focused. Your mind will then be more able to respond to suggestions (from yourself or your clinician) for beneficial changes. As you gain experience, you will find that you respond more to some inductions than others, and you can use this knowledge to design and practice inductions that are most effective for you. Although inductions are usually the first step of hypnosis or self-hypnosis, they can be beneficial in and of themselves.

Self-Hypnosis for Pain and Fatigue Management

You can learn to use self-hypnosis to experience more comfort, less pain, and more energy. The steps to achieving this goal are straightforward: (1) learn an induction to experience yourself in a relaxed and focused state and then (2) read or repeat to yourself suggestions that will help you feel more comfort. There are a wide variety of inductions you can learn, and many suggestions you could read (or repeat to yourself) that could help you achieve your goals of pain and fatigue reduction. It is likely that you will respond more positively to some of these suggestions than others, or that the suggestions you find most useful today may be different than the suggestions you will find most useful next week or several years from now.

Seven suggestions for pain and fatigue management were presented in this workbook. The clinician you are working with may also provide you with additional suggestions to use. To maximize your chances of getting the most out of self-hypnosis treatment, you would do well to try each one, and then determine the suggestion or suggestions that you respond the best to. Then repeat that suggestion (always after an induction) on a regular basis to increase the chances that the benefits will become automatic.

Self-Hypnosis for Thought and Mood Management

Hypnosis can be beneficial in ways other than just pain and fatigue management. It can also help you make changes in the way you think about pain. Because how we feel depends to a large extent on the thoughts that are going through our mind, increasing the amount of time we spend focusing on and thinking helpful and reassuring thoughts will result in substantial improvements in mood.

Importantly, thinking about and focusing on helpful thoughts following a hypnotic induction can increase the beneficial effects of those thoughts.

Three suggestions for helping you focus more on helpful thoughts were presented in the workbook. The first one encourages you to increase your ability to tolerate ambiguity—to avoid jumping to conclusions about events, and to give you time to consider the most helpful response possible. The second suggestion provides a simple strategy to increase your focus on a specific helpful thought, idea, or conclusion. The final suggestion gives you a hypnotic strategy for identifying new and potentially very useful thoughts that may be worth focusing on in future sessions.

Self-Hypnosis for Activity and Sleep Management

Pain has likely had a significant negative impact on many aspects of your life, including perhaps your ability to do what is most meaningful to you. You could choose to wait until the pain problem is cured, or at least largely resolved, before you get back to doing the things that are most important to you. However, although it is not unreasonable to anticipate that you may experience much less pain sometime in the future, what are you going to do in the meantime? If it is possible to become even more active and participate more in the activities that are meaningful starting today, you may be surprised at how your life changes for the better. You can use the self-hypnosis exercise in Chapter 9 to identify activities you wish to participate in, and then make it easier to do so.

Chronic pain may also have had a negative effect on your ability to get to sleep and stay asleep. If so, you can start to improve your sleep by making some relatively simple changes in your behavior during the day; for example, by avoiding chemicals that interfere with sleep (caffeine, nicotine, and alcohol), avoiding naps during the day, waking up and getting out of bed about the same time every day, using the bed only for sex or sleep, and developing a pre-sleep ritual that you engage in on a regular basis. You can also use one or more of your favorite self-hypnosis inductions to prepare your mind for sleep at night, or to help you get back to sleep if you wake up. Finally, you can read the self-hypnosis suggestions regarding sleep presented in Chapter 9 at some point during the day to enhance the efficacy of the self-hypnosis inductions you use at night.

As you increase the use of adaptive pain coping behaviors, engage in more activities that are most meaningful to you, and get more restful sleep at night, you should note an overall increase in the quality of your life: pain will have less of a negative impact. A common "side effect" of these changes is also a decrease in pain.

Fitting Hypnosis and Self-Hypnosis into Your Daily Life

Hypnosis

If you are working with a clinician who is providing you with hypnosis treatment, the chances are good that he or she is giving you audio recordings of the treatment sessions to listen to at home between the sessions. Even though you will be listening to these recordings on your own, they still technically meet the definition of *hypnosis* because they are recordings of your clinician providing inductions and suggestions. Still, each time you listen to these recordings, and to the extent that the suggestions are appropriate for your well-being, you can build on and enhance any gains you are making with treatment.

The research that is available supports the benefits of using audio recordings during and long after hypnosis treatment. You may find that you have a favorite recording that you choose to listen to on a regular basis. Or you may decide to listen to different recordings on different days. You will learn, based on your responses to your recordings, which option works best for you. But you should clearly consider listening to the sessions even after your face-to-face treatment with the clinician is completed.

Self-Hypnosis

Self-hypnosis involves allowing yourself to shift into a hypnotic state, usually with the aid of an induction that you respond well to, and then giving yourself a suggestion or set of suggestions. You can give yourself the suggestions by reading from a script or by simply reciting the suggestion in your mind. As you practice and gain experience, you will become more skilled at being able to give yourself suggestions during self-hypnosis.

One of the many benefits of self-hypnosis is that you can practice it any time during the day. You can give yourself a very brief 1-minute self-hypnosis suggestion (take a deep breath, hold it, let it go, and feel yourself shift into a focused state; then tell yourself a truth that is helpful and reassuring) many times during the day. You can give yourself a moderately long 5- to 10-minute session twice a day, or even a much longer session on some days. Each time you practice, you will get more skilled, and the beneficial effects of the suggestions you make will increase and amplify.

Concluding Comments

If you experience chronic pain, it is almost certainly the case that there are things that you can do so that you are able to hurt less and do more. Experts in the field of chronic pain management also agree that how well you manage your pain depends much more on what you do than on what is done to you.

One of the things that will allow you to do more and hurt less is self-hypnosis. You have already started to learn self-hypnosis skills by reading this book and practicing the inductions and suggestions that are presented. Although you can benefit from self-hypnosis by following the exercises in this workbook, the benefits you get from hypnosis will be enhanced if you work with a clinician experienced in the application of hypnotic treatments for chronic pain.

If you have not already found a clinician to work with and if you decide that you want to, it is important to choose the therapist you work with very carefully. There is no state license required to practice "hypnotherapy," so anyone can hang out a shingle or advertise and recruit potential clients. Most professionals with knowledge about hypnosis know that "hypnosis" should rarely be offered by itself. Rather, it should be offered as part of a complete pain treatment program that might (for individuals treated by licensed clinical psychologists) also include cognitive behavior therapy. Anyone offering hypnosis should have appropriate training in this approach and should also have an advanced degree (for example, a PhD or MD) and be able to offer other appropriate treatments in addition to hypnosis.

Although there is no license required to practice hypnosis, there are four reputable organizations in the United States whose members are vetted to have adequate credentials and training for using hypnosis in their clinical practice: the Society for Clinical and Experimental Hypnosis (http://www.sceh.us), the American Association of Clinical Hypnosis (http://www.asch.net), the Milton Erickson Foundation (http://www.erickson-foundation.org), and Division 30 of the American Psychological Association (http://www.apa.org/divisions/div30/homepage.html). These organizations have combined efforts to create a single Web site for individuals seeking referrals for hypnosis treatment (http://www.societiesofhypnosis.com/).

Hypnosis is not magic; it is an approach that has been demonstrated to be effective for chronic pain management, and its effects can be measured in the brain areas involved in the experience of pain. Although everyone has a unique response, almost everyone who takes the time to learn and practice self-hypnosis skills finds that he or she benefits. It is very likely that you can be one of these people.

15479117R00085

Made in the USA
Lexington, KY
30 May 2012